The CE Mark:

Understanding the Medical Device Directive

The CE Mark:

Understanding the Medical Device Directive

Les Schnoll

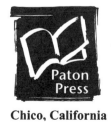

Chico, California

Most Paton Press books are available at quantity discounts when purchased in bulk. For more information, contact:

Paton Press
236 W. East Ave., Suite 261
Chico, CA 95926
(530) 342-5480
Fax (530) 342-5471
E-mail *books@patonpress.com*

01 00 99 98 97   5 4 3 2 1

Publisher .... Scott M. Paton
Director of Marketing .... Heidi M. Paton
Senior Editor .... Marion Harmon
Book Cover Design .... Angie Skillman

ISBN 0-9650445-3-X

About the Author

Les Schnoll is director of regulated industries for KPMG Quality Registrar, having joined the organization in December 1993. He is currently responsible for managing all business and technical functions and relationships for the regulated industries business segments. He has more than 25 years of experience in quality assurance/quality control, auditing, regulatory compliance, management and microbiology in medical, pharmaceutical, clinical, industrial and food areas.

Schnoll is recognized for achievements in developing quality management, regulatory compliance, auditing, sanitation, microbiological, quality assurance, material safety information and statistical process control programs. He is knowledgeable in all aspects of medical device and material, pharmaceutical, food, clinical laboratory and chemical industry objectives, as well as regulatory, packaging, safety, environmental and product stewardship programs and requirements. Schnoll is authorized by the Medical Device Agency in the United Kingdom to perform assessments to the European Union Medical Device Directive and the EN 46000 standards.

Prior to joining KPMG Quality Registrar, Schnoll was with Dow Corning Corp. as the ISO program and quality auditing manager. He was involved with the global management of all quality system registration, auditing and training activities, and has published articles on ISO 9000 for publications such as *Quality Digest, Medical Design and Material, ISO 9000 Handbook of Quality Standards and Compliance, Pharmaceutical and Medical Packaging News, Food Quality* and *Quality Progress.* Schnoll has conducted various audits and training programs in the United States, Europe, South America, Australia and Japan.

Schnoll's professional affiliations are with the American Society for Quality as a Certified Quality Engineer and a Certified Quality Auditor; American Society for Microbiology as a Specialist and a Registered Microbiologist; The International Register of Certificated Auditors as a Registered Lead Assessor; BSI Certified Tutor (Lead Assessor Training); and

American Institute of Baking as a Certified Quality Control Sanitarian. He is a member of the American Society for Quality, American Society for Microbiology, Society of Manufacturing Engineers, American National Standards Institute, Institute of Internal Auditors, The Institute of Quality Assurance, the Institute of Food Technologists, the Association for the Advancement of Medical Instrumentation, the National Association of Healthcare Quality, Strathmore's Who's Who and the Who's Who of Global Business Leaders.

Schnoll is involved with many professional activities, including the U.S. Technical Advisory Group to Technical Committee 176, International Organization for Standardization; U.S. Technical Advisory Group to Technical Committee 210, International Organization for Standardization; and the American National Standards Institute Accredited Standards Committee Z-1 on Quality Management and Quality Assurance.

Schnoll has a bachelor's of science degree in biology from Ursinus College, a master's of science in microbiology from Villanova University and a master's of business administration from Central Michigan University.

Contents

Acknowledgments

The philosophy and contents of this book stem directly from my 25 years of experience as a quality professional in the regulated industries. I have always learned something from every position that I have had in my career, and many friends and colleagues have provided me with the benefits of their insights, knowledge and understanding. However, a few people deserve special recognition.

To Joe Tsiakals at Baxter Healthcare, a quality professional in all aspects of the term, who, as a colleague and friend, provided me with opportunities to develop my knowledge of international quality standards.

To Jim Matherly at Dow Corning Corp., a friend, advisor and mentor for 15 years who always had faith in my abilities and who had the intestinal fortitude to hold people accountable for their actions and potential consequences.

Finally, to my wife, Harriet, who has always had confidence in my abilities and who met my constant howls of "Leave me alone; I'm trying to work on my book!" with love and encouragement.

Chapter 1

Introduction
The European Union and its directives

In 1985, the European Union implemented a new approach to developing standards for those products it considered critical from health and safety aspects. These new standards, which became known as directives, provide generic guidelines for those product lines and establish the basis for global marketing into the 21st century.

The documents cover about 14 product lines, from toys to electromagnetic equipment to heavy construction equipment to medical devices. Their implementation dates range from 1993 to 2007. Compliance with these directives is required to do business in the European Union, and their requirements are regulatory in nature.

In developing these documents, the European Union wanted to establish a uniform code for products sold within its member states while eliminating barriers to free movement of those goods. However, in its attempts to eliminate trade barriers for manufacturers within member states, the European Union has inadvertently created one of the best kept "secrets" for manufacturers outside the European Union.

Most organizations outside the European Union either have not heard of the directives, have no idea what is required to comply with them (or even how to get started) or are blissfully unaware of the "drop-dead" dates that mark the end of the transition periods. Many companies have heard of the CE Mark but do not know what they must accomplish before the mark can be placed on their products. Even worse, a few companies actually have begun to use the CE Mark illegally and have no clue of the penalties associated with fraudulent use of the marking.

It would be difficult to find someone who hasn't heard of the ISO 9000 series of quality system standards, compliance to which is generally voluntary. These documents clearly delineate 20 common-sense requirements that companies should follow if they want to remain in business. The ISO

9000 series, in addition to being standards for quality management, also define—and support—a profitable management system.

It's difficult to understand why, in a country like the United States, which is so widely regulated (Food and Drug Administration, Occupational Safety and Health Administration, Environmental Protection Agency, to name just a few), knowledge of and compliance to the European Union directives is so painfully lacking, especially when they define the rules that will allow manufacturers of those regulated products to continue to sell them into the European market. There are several potential answers. It could be that we just haven't heard of the requirements because they apply only to products exported to the European Union.

Perhaps the answer is that the need for compliance has not (deliberately or otherwise) been communicated to us. It may be due to other domestic pressures and regulations, coupled with our litigious society. In part, it may be due to lethargy and postponing the inevitable without realizing that time has run out. It probably is a combination of these reasons, along with a healthy dose of other issues.

Whatever the reasons, it's time to actively comply with the directives. Because the United States is not a member of the European Union, it has virtually no input into the decisions of the European Commission or the documents that it enacts. This leaves us, and a majority of countries around the world that export regulated products into the European Union, in a position where we must comply with a set of laws that have been thrust upon us. Compliance with the Medical Device Directive is not an easy task to accomplish and must be achieved by June 1998.

Overview of the Medical Device Directive

The MDD is one of the more important impending requirements that manufacturers of medical devices must meet. The directive, officially known as 93/42/EEC, is one of the more frustrating mandates to decipher and understand, making compliance more difficult than it needs to be. Unfortunately, the MDD was written by the same organization that gave us the 26,911-word treatise known as "The European Economic Community Directive for Export of Duck Eggs"!

The MDD consists of 23 articles, 12 annexes and 18 classification rules, all of which send those who must comply with the requirements scampering through a bureaucratic maze of redundancy. Reading and understanding the Food and Drug Administration's new quality system regulation is child's play compared with any attempts to digest the MDD.

The MDD is intended to harmonize standards that benefit manufacturers, users and patients, and to define the requirements for the clinical testing, design, manufacture, testing/inspection, marketing, installation and service of medical devices sold within the European Union. All medical devices sold within the European Union must conform to this directive by June 14, 1998; however, this date is the end of the phase-in period, which began on January 1, 1995.

During this transitional period, manufacturers may choose to comply with the MDD provisions and ensure that their products comply with the essential requirements, or they may choose to comply with existing member states' requirements. The disadvantage of opting to comply with current/earlier national requirements during the transition period is that manufacturers must comply with the current requirements of *all* member states in which they wish to do business.

Unfortunately, those attempting to read and understand the directives may begin to see that clarity and conciseness are mutually exclusive of the documentation of the requirements. Therefore, this book strives to present the reader with a coherent explanation of the MDD requirements and assist in providing a basis for compliance.

Chapter 2

Overview of the
Medical Device Directive
The MDD in general

The MDD's main purpose is to harmonize national controls to allow free movement of medical devices throughout the European Union and the European Free Trade Association while ensuring that all devices within the European Union are reasonably safe to use. The directive covers devices ranging from bandages and tongue depressors to knee and hip joints to X-ray equipment and CAT scanners.

The MDD covers most medical devices other than active implantable medical devices and in vitro diagnostic products; there is currently another directive (90/385/EEC) for Active Implantable Medical Devices and a proposed directive (95/C172/02) for In Vitro Diagnostics. Another directive that may come into play for manufacturers of medical devices is the Electromedical Equipment Directive (84/549/EEC). There are also European Union Good Manufacturing Practices, Good Laboratory Practices, Human Medicinal Products and Risk Assessment directives.

The MDD specifies essential requirements that manufacturers must meet before they can place any device on the market; introduces controls covering the safety, performance, specification, design, manufacture and packaging of devices; specifies requirements for assessment of clinical investigative protocols and the evaluation of any adverse incidents that occur; introduces a system of classification of devices and applies a level of control that is matched to the degree of risk inherent in the device; and empowers a competent authority to identify and designate notified bodies which check and verify that devices meet the relevant essential requirements.

Notified body intervention is not required by manufacturers of Class I medical devices unless the devices are placed on the market in a sterile condition or have a measuring function. However, manufacturers (or their authorized representatives) of Class I devices must:

- Review the device classification rules to confirm that their products fall within Class I (per MDD Annex IX).
- Check that their products meet all applicable essential requirements (MDD Annex I).
- Prepare relevant technical documentation.
- Prepare the EC Declaration of Conformity before applying the CE Mark to their products.
- Implement and maintain corrective action and vigilance procedures.
- Obtain notified body approval for sterility or metrology aspects of their devices (if applicable).
- Make all relevant documentation available for inspection on the request of the competent authority.
- Register with the competent authority.
- Notify the competent authority, in advance, of any proposals to perform a clinical investigation to demonstrate safety and performance.

Technical documentation

Medical device manufacturers must retain technical documentation that demonstrates their product's conformity with MDD requirements. They must prepare this technical documentation before preparing the EC Declaration of Conformity, and it must be available for review by the notified body and/or the competent authority.

Manufacturers should prepare the technical documentation after reviewing the essential requirements in Annex I. The documentation must cover all of the following:

- *A general description* of the product, including any variations (e.g., names, sizes, model numbers).
- *Raw material and component documentation*, including specifications (as applicable) of raw materials, drawings of components, quality control procedures and/or master patterns.
- *Intermediate product and subassembly documentation*, including specifications, appropriate drawings and master patterns, circuits, formulations, manufacturing procedures and methods, and quality control procedures.
- *Final product documentation*, including specifications, appropriate drawings and master patterns, circuits, formulations, manufacturing procedures and methods, and quality control procedures.
- *Packaging and labeling documentation*, including copies of all labels and instructions for use.

• *Design verification*, including the results of qualification tests and design calculations relevant to the product's intended use, which includes connections to other devices to allow the device to operate as intended.

• *Risk analysis results* to substantiate that any risks associated with the product's use are compatible with a high level of protection of health and safety and are weighed against the benefits to the patient and user.

• *Compliance with the essential requirements and harmonized standards*, including a list of relevant harmonized standards that have been applied to the products.

• *Clinical data*, if appropriate.

• *Records* of manufacturing, inspection and testing to show compliance with documented procedures and specifications.

Chapter 3

The Medical Device Directive Articles
Summary of requirements

Medical device manufacturers (or their authorized representatives) must be able to demonstrate compliance with the directive's applicable articles and annexes. Twenty-three articles comprise the portion of the MDD that sets the stage for compliance. This first section of the MDD provides definitions, defines the rules and routes for compliance, describes the classification of medical devices and points the reader to the document's second section: the 12 annexes that provide the detail.

Article 1: Definitions and scope

Article 1 includes the document's scope (medical devices and their accessories) as well as important definitions; it also defines those products to which the directive does not apply.

The primary definition in the MDD describes a medical device: "Any instrument, apparatus, appliance, material or other article, whether used alone or in combination, including the software necessary for its proper application, intended by the manufacturer to be used for human beings for the purpose of: diagnosis, prevention, monitoring, treatment or alleviation of disease; diagnosis, monitoring, treatment, alleviation of or compensation for an injury or handicap; investigation, replacement or modification of the anatomy or of a physiological process; control of conception; and which does not achieve its principal intended action in or on the human body by pharmacological, immunological or metabolic means, but which may be assisted in its function by such means."

The directive makes a key distinction between a medical device and a medicinal product; a product that achieves its principal action by pharmacological, immunological or metabolic means is not considered a medical device and is not subject to the MDD's provisions. Medicinal products are regulated by Directive 65/65/EEC.

The final section of Article 1 clearly defines those products regulated by other directives (or not regulated at the present time). These include:

- In vitro diagnostic devices
- Active implantable medical devices
- Medicinal products
- Cosmetic products
- Human blood, human blood products, human plasma or blood cells of human origin
- Devices that incorporate blood products, plasma or cells at the time of placing on the market
- Transplants, tissues or cells of human origin or products incorporating or derived from tissues or cells of human origin
- Transplants, tissue or cells of animal origin (unless a device is manufactured utilizing animal tissue that is rendered nonviable)
- Personal protective equipment

Article 2: Placing on the market and putting into service

Article 2 states that European Union member states are required to take any and all steps to enforce compliance with the MDD.

Article 3: Essential requirements

Article 3 specifies that all medical devices must meet the applicable essential requirements defined in Annex I; these essential requirements are basically the legal requirements for marketing medical devices in the European Union.

Article 4: Free movement, devices intended for special purposes

Member states must not impede placement of medical devices on the market, provided those devices bear the CE Mark (which means that the manufacturer has met all conformity assessment procedures defined in Article 11).

Article 4 also specifies that member states create no obstacles for custom-made devices or devices intended for clinical investigation. However, because compliance with all essential requirements cannot be demonstrated at that time for devices intended for clinical use, such devices cannot bear the CE Mark. For custom-made devices, compliance with MDD requirements is established jointly by the practitioner issuing the prescription and the manufacturer. Therefore, such devices do not bear the CE Mark.

Article 4 also says that member states cannot prohibit exhibition or demonstration of noncompliant devices at trade shows and other such exhibitions, *provided that the devices are clearly identified that they cannot be marketed or put into service until they do comply.*

The final provision is that where medical devices are subject to other directives (e.g., the Electromagnetic Compatibility Directive) in addition to the MDD, *all applicable* provisions of *all* directives must be met before the CE Mark can be affixed to the device.

Article 5: Reference to standards

Manufacturers must meet the requirements of applicable harmonized standards and guidelines (including those for EN 46001 or EN 46002). Typically, these harmonized standards are referenced or published in the *Official Journal of the European Communities.* Member states publish their national standards based on the harmonized standards in the journal. Article 5 also provides for member state recourse in the event that the member state considers that the harmonized standards do not adequately address the directive's essential requirements. Articles 6 and 7 describe these procedures.

Article 6: Committee on Standards and Technical Regulations

This section defines the activities and assistance to the Commission of the Committee on Standards and Technical Regulations in the promulgation of the directive. It provides for official opinions, drafts, position statements and meeting minutes.

Article 7: Committee on Medical Devices

Article 7 defines the activities and assistance to the Commission of the Committee on Medical Devices in the promulgation of the directive. It provides for official opinions, drafts, position statements and meeting minutes.

Article 8: Safeguard clause

This article provides member states with the authority to restrict or prohibit placement or withdraw devices for failure of the manufacturer to meet the essential requirements, for incorrect application of the standards referenced in Article 5 and/or for shortcomings in the standards themselves. The actions of the member states are reviewed by the Commission to determine if they are justified and what, if any, further actions either the Commission or member states require.

Article 9: Classification

Article 9 classifies medical devices into classes I, IIa, IIb and III in accordance with MDD Annex IX. It also states that in the event of a classification dispute between the manufacturer and the notified body, the decision must be referred to the competent authority (the organization that accredits the notified body) for resolution. (Chapter 5 provides more detailed information on device classification.)

Article 10: Information on incidents occurring following placing of devices on the market

This section describes the necessary steps that member states and the manufacturer must take in the event of a serious injury or death in which the medical device was involved. This is basically the directive's "recall clause" and is similar to the requirements of the Medical Device Reporting Regulation (21 CFR 803).

Article 11: Conformity assessment procedures

Article 11 defines the conformity assessment procedures summarized earlier. It also describes conformity requirements for custom-made devices and devices intended for clinical investigations.

For Class I devices (other than those that are custom-made or intended for clinical investigations), the manufacturer may declare that the product complies with the MDD's essential requirements (Annex VII), prepare technical documentation and affix the CE Mark. The manufacturer (or its authorized representative) must register its activities with the competent authority of the member country in which its registered business is located. A notified body does not need to be engaged for these activities. The exceptions to this procedure are for Class I devices supplied in a sterile condition or that have a measuring function. In such cases, the notified body must examine the manufacturing process with respect to sterility and/ or measuring function.

For Class IIa devices (other than those that are custom-made or intended for clinical investigation), the manufacturer has two options. The first option is for Full Quality Assurance System (Annex II, except for Section 4) assessment; the second option is for the EC Declaration of Conformity (defined in Annex VII) coupled with either the procedure relating to EC Verification (Annex IV), the EC Declaration of Conformity (Production Quality Assurance, Annex V) or the EC Declaration of Conformity (Product Quality Assurance, Annex VI).

For Class IIb devices (other than those that are custom-made or intended for clinical investigation), the manufacturer has two options. The first choice is for assessment of the Full Quality Assurance System (Annex II, except for Section 4); the second choice is for the EC Type-Examination (Annex III) coupled with either the procedure relating to EC Verification (Annex IV), the EC Declaration of Conformity (Production Quality Assurance, Annex V) or the EC Declaration of Conformity (Product Quality Assurance, Annex VI).

For Class III devices (other than those that are custom-made or intended for clinical investigation), the manufacturer also has two options for conformity. The first is for assessment of the Full Quality Assurance System (Annex II); the second is for the EC Type-Examination (Annex III), coupled with either the procedure relating to EC Verification (Annex IV) or the EC Declaration of Conformity (Production Quality Assurance, Annex V).

Annex VIII describes requirements for custom-made devices; Annex X describes requirements for devices intended for clinical investigation.

Table 3.1 summarizes the Conformity Assessment Procedures defined in the MDD. Chapter 7 provides more detailed information on conformity assessment procedures.

Article 12: Particular procedure for systems and procedure packs

Article 12 defines requirements to be met for assembly or sterilization of devices that bear the CE Mark. Such activities require verification of mutual compatibility, appropriate packaging and appropriate controls and inspections. Sterilization requires compliance with the procedures in annexes IV, V or VI.

Where the conditions described in Article 12 cannot be met, each component must be treated as a device in its own right and subjected to the provisions in Article 11.

Article 13: Decisions regarding classification, derogation clause

This section provides for a decision of the application of the classification rules defined in Annex IX specific to classification of a device or family of devices. This provision comes into play when a member state considers that:

• Application of the classification rules requires a decision with regard to the classification of a particular device or family of devices.

• A device or family of devices should be classified in another class.

• The conformity of a device or family of devices should be established.

In any of the above events, the member state must submit a substantiated request to the Commission seeking action and resolution. The Commission will then publish its actions and decisions in the *Official Journal of the European Communities*.

Article 14: Registration of persons responsible for placing devices on the market

Article 14 defines the requirements for registration of responsible persons (or designated individuals) who place devices on the market within the European Union. The responsible person (who can be the authorized representative) *must* have a registered business in a member state. The competent authority must be notified of the address of the registered place of business and the descriptions/categories of the devices concerned.

Article 15: Clinical investigation

This article describes the requirements for devices intended for clinical investigations (primarily compliance with annexes VIII and X) and notification of the competent authorities in the member states in which the investigations are conducted. This section also provides for time periods during which certain activities must be completed. The manufacturer (or authorized representative) must maintain appropriate documentation and provide it to the competent authority upon request. An ethics committee may play a role in evaluating the investigation plan and its acceptability relative to the roles of patient health and ethical considerations.

Article 16: Notified bodies

Article 16 defines identification and responsibilities of notified bodies. It provides for notification of the Commission by the member states of those organizations designated as notified bodies to perform the tasks for which they have been designated, as well as those tasks pertaining to Article 11. The Commission then assigns identification numbers to those notified bodies. Once so designated, the notified body must document its assessment and verification procedures. A member state may withdraw authority from any notified body if it finds that the notified body can no longer meet the defined criteria.

Article 17: CE marking

Article 17 describes the requirements for CE marking (primarily identified in Annex XII), accompanied by the identification number of the notified body responsible for implementing the procedures defined in annexes II, IV, V and VI. Devices, other than custom-made devices or devices intended for clinical investigation, that comply with the essential requirements must bear the CE Mark of conformity.

Article 18: Wrongly affixed CE marking

Article 18 articulates the penalties for wrongly affixing the CE Mark to medical devices. The CE Mark may be considered wrongly affixed if a member state establishes that the mark has been unduly placed. Once a member state determines such, the manufacturer or authorized representative must correct the violation under the conditions imposed by the member state. If the infringement continues, the member state may prohibit the manufacturer (or authorized representative) from placing the medical device on the market in the future.

Article 19: Decision in respect of refusal or restriction

Article 19 describes the appeal procedures a medical device manufacturer must follow in the event that its product is restricted or refused placement within the European Union.

Article 20: Confidentiality

Article 20 binds member states to confidentiality with regard to all information obtained in promulgating the directive.

Article 21: Repeal and amendment of directives

Article 21 repeals and/or amends several previously ratified directives based on the issuance of 93/42/EEC.

Table 3.1: Conformity Assessment Annexes

Class	Conformity Assessment Annexes
I	I and VII
I (Sterile)	I and (as appropriate) IV, V, VI, VII
I (Measuring)	I and (as appropriate) IV, V, VI, VII
IIa	I and II (except Section 4) of VII coupled with IV, V, VI (as appropriate)
IIb	I and II (except Section 4) or III coupled with IV, V, VI (as appropriate)
III	I and II or III coupled with IV, V (as appropriate)

Article 22: Implementation and transitional provisions

Article 22 describes the MDD's implementation and transition periods.

Article 23: Adoption of the Medical Device Directive

Article 23 defines and authorizes the MDD, effective June 14, 1993.

Chapter 4

The Medical Device Directive Annexes
Meeting the requirements

Twelve annexes comprise this section of the MDD—they define the compliance requirements. The annexes provide the rules, requirements and assessment routes companies must follow. The annexes are complex and wordy, and do not describe a clear path to reach the finish line—CE marking of the medical device. The following attempts to clarify the annexes:

Annex I: The Essential Requirements

This is the most important section of the MDD because the essential requirements are the legal requirements that must be met by the end of the transition period (June 14, 1998). These requirements divide into six general requirements and eight design and construction requirements.

Minimum essential requirements for the design and manufacture of medical devices ensure the protection of the health and safety of patients, users and third parties. They stipulate that safety principles should be integral to product design and that the product should be suitable for its intended purpose.

General requirements. The general requirements of Annex I state that:
• The devices must be designed and manufactured in such a way that, when used under the conditions and purposes intended, they will not compromise the health or safety of patients, users or other personnel.
• Safety principles must be utilized for the design and construction, and they should include state-of-the-art technologies.
• The devices must meet all claimed performance criteria.
• The devices must continue to function as intended, without compromising safety or health, when subjected to normal conditions of use.
• The device must not be adversely affected during defined transport and storage conditions.

• Any undesirable side effects must constitute an acceptable risk when weighed against intended performance.

Design and construction requirements. These detailed requirements of Annex I define a variety of provisions to be met (as applicable), including:
• Chemical, physical and biological properties
• Infection and microbial contamination
• Construction and environmental properties
• Properties for devices with a measuring function
• Protection against radiation
• Protection against electrical, mechanical, thermal risks, energy supplies or energy substances
• Labeling requirements and instructions for use
• If applicable, demonstration of conformance with essential requirements based on clinical data

Chapter 6 provides additional details on the essential requirements.

Annex II: EC Declaration of Conformity (Full quality assurance system)

Under this conformity assessment route, once the manufacturer has obtained full quality system registration (including the applicable EN 46000 standard), it is entitled to self-declare. This is the most commonly used conformity route and makes the most sense for those organizations that have registered quality systems. Specifics of Annex II include:
• The manufacturer's quality system must be registered to the applicable ISO 9000 and EN 46000 standards, and be subject to routine surveillance assessments. This includes an application for assessment of the quality system to/by a notified body and fulfilling an obligation to notify the competent authorities of any instance of serious injury or death from any of its medical devices. The application must include an adequate description of the manufacturer's quality objectives, business organization, procedures for monitoring and verifying product design, inspection and testing techniques during the manufacturing stages, and final release/approval criteria.
• The manufacturer must inform the notified body that approved the quality system of any planned *substantial* changes to its quality system.
• The manufacturer must declare its conformity to the MDD and affix the CE Mark in compliance with Article 17 and Annex XII.
• For Class III products, the manufacturer's technical files/design dos-

siers must be examined by the notified body to determine compliance with the essential requirements.

* Changes to the design must be approved by the notified body.
* The manufacturer is required to maintain its declarations of conformity for at least five years after the last product has been manufactured.

Annex III: EC Type-Examination

With EC type-examination, a notified body ascertains and certifies that a representative sample of the production covered meets the applicable provisions of the directive. This conformity assessment route requires the notified body to test and evaluate a representative sample of the device to ensure that the device complies fully with the MDD's applicable requirements and the appropriate technical standards. When the Annex III route is used, it is in conjunction with the procedures defined in Annex IV or Annex V.

Annex IV: EC Verification

With EC verification, the manufacturer (or authorized representative established within the European Union) ensures and declares that the products which have been subject to the procedures meet the directive's applicable requirements. The EC verification conformity assessment route requires the manufacturer of the medical device (or authorized agent) to declare that the product complies with all appropriate MDD requirements and applicable technical specifications.

Compliance is based on examinations and tests performed by the notified body. The notified body may, at its discretion, evaluate 100 percent of the devices or use rational statistical sampling methods. If statistical (batch) sampling is utilized, random samples must be taken from each batch manufactured.

If the batch is accepted, all products in the batch may be placed on the market (except those in the sample that failed); if the batch is rejected, the notified body must take appropriate measures to prevent the batch from being placed on the market. If there is a trend of frequent batch rejection, the notified body may ultimately suspend the statistical verification process and revert to 100-percent examination and testing.

Sampling and statistical control of product is based on attribute testing, requiring a sampling system that ensures a limited quantity corresponding to a probability of acceptance of 5 percent, with a nonconformity percentage of between 3 percent and 7 percent.

Annex V: EC Declaration of Conformity
(Production quality assurance)

Under this assessment process, the manufacturer must obtain a production-quality assurance registration (production and final testing) in accordance with the appropriate EN 46000 standard. Compliance with Annex V must be coupled with the procedures defined in either Annex III or Annex VII (depending upon product classification). The manufacturer must ensure the application of the quality system approved for the manufacture of the devices concerned and perform final inspection and testing, and is subject to surveillance by the notified body. The manufacturer also must affix the CE Mark to the products and prepare a written declaration of conformity for a specified number of units manufactured.

Annex VI: EC Declaration of Conformity
(Product quality assurance)

Under this assessment process, the manufacturer must obtain a product-quality assurance registration (final testing only) in accordance with the appropriate EN 46000 standard. Compliance with Annex V must be coupled with the procedures defined in either Annex III or Annex VII (depending upon product classification). The manufacturer must ensure the application of the quality system approved for final inspection and testing of the product, and is subject to surveillance by the notified body. The manufacturer also must affix the CE Mark to the products and prepare a written declaration of conformity for a specified number of units manufactured.

Annex VII: EC Declaration of Conformity

With EC declaration of conformity, the manufacturer (or authorized representative established within the European Union) fulfills the obligations imposed by the directive and declares such. Compliance with this assessment route requires that the manufacturer of the medical device prepare the appropriate technical documentation to demonstrate full compliance with the requirements of the directive and associated technical standards. The technical documentation should include:

- A general description of the product
- Design drawings, diagrams, schematics
- Product descriptions and explanations
- Results of risk analysis
- A listing of applicable standards
- A description of the sterilization process (sterile products only)

- Results of design calculations and inspections
- Test and inspection reports (and clinical data, if applicable) to support compliance with the MDD
- Labeling and instructions for use

The manufacturer must also institute and maintain a systematic procedure for review of devices in the postproduction phase and must implement appropriate means to apply any necessary corrective actions based on the review and in association with risks related to the product.

Annex VIII: Statement Concerning Devices for Special Purposes

The processes and procedures defined in Annex VIII apply to custom-made devices or devices designed for clinical investigation. The manufacturer must provide specific documentation relative to the product's intended use.

For custom-made devices, this information includes:
- Product identification information and data
- A statement declaring that the device is intended for use by a specific patient, as well as the identification of the patient
- The name of the medical practitioner or authorized individual associated with the device
- A listing of features of the device specified in the prescription
- A statement that the device conforms to the essential requirements in Annex I and, where applicable, identification of any essential requirements that have not been met

For devices intended for clinical investigation, this section includes similar information, but is more explicitly defined in Annex X.

Annex IX: Classification Criteria

This portion of the MDD includes three general sections: definitions, procedures for implementing rules and the classification rules themselves. Several definitions applicable to device classification are those for duration (transient, short-term, long-term) and device types (invasive device, surgically invasive device, implantable device, active medical device, etc.).

The classification section is rather vague and takes some skill to properly classify the device. The latest revision of the MDD includes a supplement on classification rules that is more explicit, includes several examples and attempts to streamline and simplify the process.

Annex X: Clinical Evaluation

This section provides details on requirements pertinent to devices intended for clinical investigation. These mandates include compilation of data, statements of confidentiality, and documentation of:
• Product identification information and data
• Clinical investigation plan, including the purpose, grounds, scope and number of devices
• The names of the medical practitioners and/or authorized individuals associated with the investigation
• The identification of the institution responsible for the investigation
• The location, commencement dates and scheduled duration of the investigation
• A statement that the investigation will be performed in accordance with the ethical requirements defined in the Helsinki Declaration
• A statement that the device conforms to the essential requirements in Annex I and that every precaution has been taken to protect the health and safety of the patients

Annex XI: Criteria to Be Met for the Designation of Notified Bodies

This section defines the selection criteria, conduct and responsibilities of those organizations designated as notified bodies. Notified bodies must be accredited by competent authorities. (Chapter 9 provides additional information regarding notified bodies.)

Annex XII: CE Marking of Conformity

This requirement defines the physical dimensions and appearance of the CE Mark.

Chapter 5

Medical Device Classification
Risk-assessment criteria

It would be extremely difficult to justify subjecting all medical devices to the same rigorous conformity assessment procedures. Rationally, then, a graduated system of controls corresponding to potential hazards would be more appropriate. Such classification should be based on potential hazards related to the device's intended use, possible device failures, the device's duration of contact with the human body, the device's degree of invasiveness and whether the device provides a local or systemic effect on the body.

As mentioned previously, Article 9 places all medical devices into one of four classes of increasing risk to the patient according to their properties, function and intended purpose. The level of control is proportionate to the level of risk to ensure protection of patient health. This device classification is as follows:

• *Class I devices* pose a low risk to the patient and, except for sterile products or measuring devices, can be self-certified by the manufacturer. Generally speaking, these devices do not enter into contact or interact with the body.

• *Class IIa devices* pose a medium risk and may require assessed quality systems to the ISO 9000/EN 46000 standards. Generally speaking, these devices are invasive in their interaction with the human body, but the invasion methods are limited to natural body orifices. The category may also include therapeutic devices used in diagnosis or in wound management.

• *Class IIb devices* pose a medium risk and may require assessed quality systems to the ISO 9000/EN 46000 standards; third-party certification is required. Generally speaking, these devices either are partially or totally implantable within the human body and may modify the biological or chemical composition of body fluids.

• *Class III devices* pose high risk and require design/clinical trial reviews, product certification and an assessed quality system. All third-party product and system certification must be conducted by a European notified body (or designee through formal agreement). Generally speaking, these devices affect the functioning of vital organs and/or life support systems.

Annex IX includes three general sections: definitions, procedures for implementing rules and the classification rules themselves. Five implementing rules and 18 classification rules used to classify medical devices require interpretation because they contain no clear-cut categories.

Definitions

The glossary contains the definitions in Annex IX; however, because the duration of use of the medical device is critical to determining the device classification, this chapter also includes those definitions.

The time period that the device performs its intended function affects classification. Three definitions for duration of use apply to the directive: *transient* (normally intended for continuous use for less than 60 minutes), *short-term* (normally intended for continuous use for not more than 30 days) and *long-term* (normally intended for continuous use for more than 30 days).

Implementing rules

Five implementing rules set the ground rules for further classification of the medical device. These are probably the most clearly defined rules and do not require a degree in linguistics to allow for their interpretation.
- *Rule 1*. The classification must be based on the device's intended purpose. This is very simple: The risk level and, consequently, the classification of the medical device must be based on how the device is intended to be used.
- *Rule 2*. If the medical device is intended to be used in conjunction with another medical device, the classification of each device must be performed separately. This rule also specifies that accessories be classified separately from any devices. In short, if a medical device system includes tubing (an accessory), a plasma centrifuge (device one) and a cell counter (device two), each component must be classified separately and not as a system.
- *Rule 3*. If any software drives or influences a medical device, that software automatically falls under the same classification as the medical device. Therefore, the software that runs a cerebrovascular monitoring system falls into the same class as the hardware itself.
- *Rule 4*. If the medical device is not intended to be used solely or principally in a specific area of the body, the medical device must be classified

on the basis of its most critical use. For example, if a device may be used to stimulate nerves on the hand, leg or face, it must be classified for its intended use on or in the most stringent or critical area (in this example, the face).
• *Rule 5.* If several rules apply to the same medical device, the most stringent rules resulting in the higher classification of the medical devices must be applied. For example, if a suture can be used on both skin and blood vessels, the higher classification for the blood vessels must be used for the generic suture. To avoid the higher classification, a suture intended to be used only on the skin must state the intended use on the labeling.

Classification rules

Eighteen classification rules place the medical device into one of the four device classifications described above. These are the least clearly defined rules and require a great deal of experience to understand and apply correctly; interpretation may become an issue due to the language used.

The rules are listed below. Editorial privilege has been taken to correct grammar and provide for easier understanding of the requirements. Under each rule are additional clarification and medical device examples. (Appendixes 5 through 7 assist further in determining if a medical device is noninvasive, invasive or active.)

Rule 1—All noninvasive devices are in Class I unless one of the following rules applies.

Rule subtitle: Devices that contact intact skin only or do not touch the patient

Interpretation: This baseline general rule applies to devices that only come into contact with intact skin or do not touch the patient. The key term from the perspective of the directive is noninvasive. The caveat is that the manufacturer must review the remaining 17 rules to see if any of them apply.

Examples:
• Body-liquid collection devices intended to be used in a manner that makes a return flow unlikely (e.g., wound drainage devices, urine collection bottles, incontinence pads, ostomy pouches)
• Devices intended to immobilize the body and/or apply force or compression (e.g., plaster of Paris, cervical collars, compression hosiery, gravity traction devices)
• Devices intended for external patient support (e.g., hospital beds, stretchers, wheelchairs)

• Miscellaneous devices such as corrective lenses and frames, stethoscopes, incision drapes and conductive gels

Rule 2—All noninvasive devices intended for channeling or storing blood, body liquids or tissues, liquids or gases for the purpose of eventual infusion, administration or introduction into the body are in Class IIa if they are connected to an active medical device of Class IIa or higher, if they are intended for use in storing or channeling blood or other body fluids, or if they are used for storing organs, parts of organs or body tissues.

In all other cases, they are in Class I.

Rule subtitle: Channeling or storing devices

Interpretation: These devices are different from noncontact devices in Rule 1 because they may be indirectly invasive. During their intended use, they channel or store materials that eventually will be delivered into the human body and are generally used in transfusion, infusion and anesthesia delivery.

Examples in Class I:
• Devices intended to provide a simple gravity-feed channeling function (e.g., tubing used for intravenous drips)
• Devices intended to be used for temporary storage (e.g., cups and spoons used to administer medication)

Examples in Class IIa:
• Devices intended to be used as channels in active drug-delivery systems (e.g., infusion pump tubing)
• Devices used for channeling or storage of gases (e.g., anesthesia breathing circuits)
• Devices intended to channel blood (e.g., in transfusions)
• Devices intended for temporary organ storage and transportation
• Devices intended for long-term storage of biological substances and tissues (e.g., sperm, ova, corneas)

Rule 3—All noninvasive devices intended for modifying the biological or chemical composition of blood, other body liquids or other liquids intended for infusion into the body are in Class IIb.

If the treatment consists of filtration, centrifugation or exchanges of gas or heat, they are in Class IIa.

Rule subtitle: Devices that modify biological or chemical composition

Interpretation: This rule covers those devices that are indirectly invasive and treat or modify substances that will be delivered into the body. Generally speaking, Rule 3 covers the components of extracorporeal circulation sets, dialysis systems and autotransfusion systems.

Examples in Class IIa:
- Equipment for particulate filtration of blood
- Blood centrifuges
- Gas exchange equipment
- Blood warming/cooling systems

Examples in Class IIb:
- Hemodialyzers
- Blood cell separation systems

Rule 4—All noninvasive devices that come into contact with injured skin are in Class I if they are intended to be used as a mechanical barrier, for compression or for absorption of exudates.

They are in Class IIb if they are intended to be used primarily with wounds that have breached the dermis and can only heal by secondary intent.

They are in Class IIa in all other cases, including devices principally intended to manage the microenvironment of a wound.

Rule subtitle: Injured skin contact devices

Interpretation: This rule primarily pertains to wound dressings. The manufacturer's intended use is paramount in determining the device's classification.

Class I devices are primary dressings for simple wounds that generally act as a barrier and/or promote the healing process. These dressings typically absorb wound exudates and are frequently applied using adhesive bandages.

Class IIa devices have specific properties intended to aid in the healing process by controlling the level of moisture at the wound and control the microenvironment (humidity, temperature, oxygen level).

Class IIb devices are intended to be used with severe wounds that have breached the dermis and can be healed only by secondary intent.

Examples in Class I: Gauze and adhesive dressings

Examples in Class IIa: Adhesives for topical use

Examples in Class IIb: Dressings for chronic ulcerated wounds, severe burns, decubitus wounds

Rule 5—All invasive devices with respect to body orifices, other than surgically invasive devices that are not intended for connection to an active medical device, are in Class I if they are intended for transient use.

Such devices are in Class IIa if they are intended for short-term use.

If they are used in the oral cavity as far as the pharynx, in an ear canal up to the eardrum or in a nasal cavity, they are in Class I.

Such devices are in Class IIb if they are intended for long-term use.

If they are used in the oral cavity as far as the pharynx, in an ear canal up to the eardrum or in a nasal cavity and are not likely to be absorbed by mucus, they are in Class IIa.

All invasive devices with respect to body orifices, other than surgically invasive devices, intended for connection to an active medical device in Class IIa or higher are in Class IIa.

Rule subtitle: Body orifice invasive devices

Interpretation: This rule covers those devices that are invasive through a natural body orifice (ear, mouth, nose, eye, anus, urethra, vagina, penis) as well as those invasive through a permanent artificial orifice (e.g., a stoma). Medical devices covered by Rule 5 are generally diagnostic and therapeutic instruments used by specialists (e.g., ophthalmologists, urologists, proctologists, gynecologists, dentists and ENT specialists).

Examples in Class I: Handheld dental mirrors, dental impression materials, stomach tubes, dental instruments, enemas, examination gloves, dentures, hearing aid inserts

Examples in Class IIa: Contact lenses, urinary catheters, tracheotomy tubes, orthodontic wire, nasopharyngeal airways

Example in Class IIb: Urethral stents

Rule 6—All surgically invasive devices intended for transient use are in Class IIa.

Devices intended specifically to diagnose, monitor or correct a defect of the heart or of the central circulatory system through direct contact with those parts of the body are in Class III.

Reusable surgical instruments are in Class I.

Devices intended to have a biological effect or to be wholly absorbed are in Class IIb.

Those intended to supply energy in the form of ionizing radiation are in Class IIb.

Devices intended to administer medication by means of a delivery system in a manner that is potentially hazardous (taking account of the mode of application) are in Class IIb.

Rule subtitle: Transient surgically invasive devices

Interpretation: This rule addresses three basic groups of medical devices that are transient in their use; these devices include those that create a conduit through the skin (e.g., needles), surgical instruments (e.g., scalpels) and catheters.

Examples in Class I: Scalpels, drill bits, retractors, surgical saws

Examples in Class IIa: Suture needles, syringe needles, lances

Example in Class IIb: Insulin pens

Example in Class III: Cardiovascular catheters

Rule 7—All surgically invasive devices intended for short-term use are in Class IIa.

If they are intended either specifically to diagnose, monitor or correct a defect of the heart or of the central circulatory system through direct contact with those parts of the body, they are in Class III.

If they are intended specifically for use in direct contact with the central nervous system, they are in Class III.

If they are intended to supply energy in the form of ionizing radiation, they are in Class IIb.

If they are intended to have a biological effect or to be wholly absorbed, they are in Class III.

If they are intended to undergo chemical change in the body, except if the devices are placed in the teeth or to administer medication, they are in Class IIb.

Rule subtitle: Short-term surgically invasive devices

Interpretation: This rule covers those medical devices used during surgery or for postoperative care.

Examples in Class IIa:
• Drainage catheters
• Clamps
• Cannulae
• Needles
• Skin-closure devices

Examples in Class IIb:
• Ionizing radiation (e.g., brachytherapy devices)
• Chemical changes (e.g., adhesives)

Examples in Class III:
- Contact with heart or CCS (e.g., cardiovascular catheters)
- Contact with CNS (e.g., neurological catheters, cortical electrodes)
- Biological effect/absorbed (e.g., absorbable sutures, biological adhesives)

Rule 8—All implantable devices and long-term surgically invasive devices are in Class IIb.

Devices intended to be placed in the teeth are in Class IIa.

Those intended to be used in direct contact with the heart, the central circulatory system or the central nervous system are in Class III.

Devices intended to have a biological effect or to be wholly absorbed are in Class III.

Those intended to undergo chemical change in the body, except if the devices are placed in the teeth or to administer medication, are in Class III.

Rule subtitle: Long-term surgically invasive devices

Interpretation: This rule applies to soft tissue, orthopedic, ophthalmic and cardiovascular implants.

Examples in Class IIa:
- Bridges
- Crowns
- Dental alloys

Examples in Class IIb:
- Prosthetic joints (e.g., joint replacements, ligaments, shunts, stents, nails, plates)
- Intraocular lenses
- Internal closure devices
- Tissue augmentation implants
- Vascular grafts
- Absorbable sutures
- Bone cement

Examples in Class III:
- Contact with heart, CNS, CCS (e.g., prosthetic heart valves, aneurysm clips, vascular prostheses, spinal and vascular stents, cardiovascular sutures, hydrocephalic shunts)
- Biological effect/absorbed (e.g., absorbable sutures and implants covered with a biologically active coating, adhesives)
- Chemical changes (e.g., nonactive drug-delivery systems)

Rule 9—All active therapeutic devices intended to administer or exchange energy are in Class IIa.

If their characteristics are such that they may administer or exchange energy to or from the human body in a potentially hazardous way, taking into account the nature, density and site of application of the energy, they are in Class IIb.

All active devices intended to control or monitor the performance of active therapeutic devices in Class IIb or intended to directly influence the performance of such devices are in Class IIb.

Rule subtitle: Active therapeutic devices

Interpretation: This rule includes medical devices that are typically electrical equipment used in surgery. Also included are devices for specialized treatment (such as radiation treatment) and stimulation (such as TENS devices).

Examples in Class IIa:
- Electrical and magnetic energy (e.g., muscle stimulators, TENS devices)
- Thermal energy (e.g., warming blankets, cryosurgery equipment)
- Kinetic energy (e.g., dermatomes)
- Light (e.g., lasers for skin treatment, phototherapy devices)
- Sound (e.g., hearing aids)

Examples in Class IIb:
- Electrical energy (e.g., electrosurgical generators, defibrillators, external pacemakers, electrocautery equipment)
- Thermal energy (e.g., neonatal incubators, blood warmers)
- Kinetic energy (e.g., lung ventilators)
- Light (e.g., surgical lasers)
- Sound (e.g., lithotriptors)
- Ionizing radiation (e.g., linear accelerators)

Rule 10—Active devices intended for diagnosis are in Class IIa.

If the devices are intended to supply energy that will be absorbed by the human body, except for devices used to illuminate the patient's body in the visible spectrum, they are in Class IIa.

Devices intended to image in vivo distribution of radiopharmaceuticals are in Class IIa.

Those intended to allow direct diagnosis or monitoring of vital physiological processes are in Class IIa.

If the devices are specifically intended to monitor vital physiological parameters where the nature of variability could result in immediate danger to the patient (e.g., variation in cardiac performance, respiration, CNS activity), they are in Class IIb.

Active devices intended to emit ionizing radiation and intended for diagnostic and therapeutic interventional radiology, including devices that control or monitor such devices or which directly influence their performance, are in Class IIb.

Rule subtitle: Active diagnostic devices

Interpretation: This rule covers a broad spectrum of equipment used in therapeutic and diagnostic radiology, ultrasound diagnosis and the acquisition of physiological signals.

Examples in Class IIa:
• Energy absorption (e.g., nuclear magnetic resonance equipment, ultrasound imaging systems)
• Radiopharmaceutical imaging (e.g., gamma camera)
• Physiological diagnosis and monitoring (e.g., electrocardiographs, electroencephalographs)

Examples in Class IIb:
• Vital physiological monitoring (e.g., apnea monitors, biological sensors, intensive care monitoring systems)
• Ionizing radiation (e.g., X-ray equipment, CAT scanners)

Rule 11—All active devices intended to administer and/or remove medicines, body fluids or other substances to or from the body are in Class IIa.

If this activity is performed in a manner that is potentially hazardous, taking into account the nature of the substances involved, the portion of the body concerned and mode of application, the device is in Class IIb.

Rule subtitle: Active delivery system devices

Interpretation: This rule covers drug-delivery systems and anesthesia equipment, as well as equipment used in the removal of fluids from the body.

Examples in Class IIa: Suction equipment, feeding pumps

Examples in Class IIb: Infusion pumps, ventilators, dialysis equipment, anesthesia equipment, blood pumps for heart-lung machines

Rule 12—All other active devices are in Class I.

Rule subtitle: Other active devices

Interpretation: This rule is considered the "fall-back" rule, covering all

other active medical devices not covered in rules 9 through 11.
Examples: Surgical microscopes, examination lights

Rule 13—All devices incorporating, as an integral part, a substance that, if used separately, can be considered to be a medicinal product and that is likely to act on the human body with action ancillary to that of the devices are in Class III.
Rule subtitle: Devices incorporating a medicinal substance
Interpretation: This rule covers a combination of medical devices that contain medicinal substances incorporated into the device for the purpose of assisting in the functioning of the device; the primary function of the device does *not* rely on the effect of the medicinal substance. If, however, the medical device *does* rely on the pharmacological agent, the product is not considered a device and is not included in the scope of the MDD.
Examples: Antibiotic bone cement and condoms containing spermicide

Rule 14—All devices used for contraception or the prevention of the transmission of sexually transmitted diseases are in Class IIb.
Implantable or long-term invasive devices are in Class III.
Rule subtitle: Contraception and sexually transmitted diseases
Interpretation: This rule covers those devices intended to be used for contraception and the prevention of sexually transmitted diseases. In some cases (e.g., condoms), the device may be intended to provide both functions.
Examples in Class IIb: Condoms, diaphragms
Examples in Class III: Intrauterine devices

Rule 15—All devices intended specifically to be used for disinfecting, cleaning, rinsing or hydrating contact lenses are in Class IIb.
All devices intended specifically to be used for disinfecting medical devices are in Class IIa.
Rule subtitle: Disinfecting, cleaning and rinsing devices
Interpretation: This rule addresses contact lens fluids and substances used to disinfect medical devices. This rule does *not* apply to products intended to clean medical devices, other than contact lenses, by means of physical action.
Examples in Class IIb: Contact lens solutions
Examples in Class IIa: Disinfectants intended for wet sterilization of proctoscopes

Rule 16—Nonactive devices specifically intended for recording of X-ray diagnostic images are in Class IIa.

Rule subtitle: X-ray films

Interpretation: This rule applies to nonactive devices specifically intended to record X-ray diagnostic images.

Example: X-ray film

Rule 17—All devices manufactured utilizing animal tissues or derivatives rendered nonviable, except if they are intended to come into contact with intact skin only, are in Class III.

Rule subtitle: Devices utilizing animal tissues/derivatives

Interpretation: This rule includes devices that are made of or contain animal tissues that have been rendered nonviable, i.e., where there is no longer any cellular metabolic activity. Any devices that contain human tissue and/or viable animal tissue are excluded from the scope of the MDD.

Examples: Biological heart valves, porcine xenograft dressings, collagen dressings/implants

Rule 18—Blood bags are in Class IIb.

Rule subtitle: Blood bags

Interpretation: This special rule covers only blood bags.

Example: Blood bags (including those coated with an anticoagulant)

Now that the classification rules have been introduced and interpreted, it would be useful to classify an example of a medical device. Rather than to use a device that is very simple and would fall into Class I or one that is extremely complex that may fall into Class III, let's use an ultrasound stethoscope for our review.

Using the classification rules, the reader should be able to conclude that the device is a Class IIa device, is an active device because it introduces ultrasonic energy into the body and is classified using Rule 10 (intended for diagnosis and intended to supply energy that will be absorbed by the human body). It is also a noninvasive device and is considered to be transient.

A second (verifying) method that will bring the reader to the same conclusion is by using the decision trees in appendixes 5 and 6. Beginning with the noninvasive flowchart (Appendix 5) and using the definition for an active medical device in the directive, the reader would be led to the active device flowchart (Appendix 6). Following the chart down and to the right, the reader would be advised that the device falls into Class IIa.

Chapter 6

Essential Requirements
The legal requirements

Chapter 2 provides an overview of the essential requirements in Annex I of the MDD. However, Annex I contains a tremendous amount of detail, and *all* of the listed requirements in *each* category must be addressed and objective evidence provided to the notified body—even if the response to a particular area is "not applicable."

The essential requirements are relatively forthright, requiring no significant interpretation. In some cases, compliance with other European Union directives may be required and are so defined in Appendix I. Complying with the essential requirements is definitely essential. These are the *legal* requirements to place medical devices on the market in the European Union and, as found in other areas of the MDD, failure to comply can result in significant penalties to the manufacturer or authorized representative.

The remainder of this chapter lists the essential requirements. The author has taken the liberty of structuring this list in the form of a "template" that the reader can use to respond to these qualifying factors and to provide a summary or catalog of objective evidence to the notified body assessing compliance of the medical device. *[Note: Electronic or printed copies of this template can be obtained from the publisher.]*

Medical Device Directive (93/42/EEC)
Annex I—Essential Requirements
Medical Device:_____
Page ____ of ____

I. General Requirements

1. The devices must be designed and manufactured in such a way that, when used under the conditions and for the purposes intended, they will not compromise the clinical condition or the safety of patients, or the safety and health of users or, where applicable, other persons, provided that any risks which may be associated with their use constitute acceptable risks when weighed against the benefits to the patient and are compatible with a high level of protection of health and safety.

Reply:

2. The solutions adopted by the manufacturer for the design and construction of the devices must conform to safety principles, taking account of the generally acknowledged state of the art. In selecting the most appropriate solutions, the manufacturer must apply the following principles in the following order:
   • eliminate or reduce risks as far as possible (inherently safe design and construction),
   • where appropriate, take adequate protection measures including alarms if necessary, in relation to risks that cannot be eliminated,
   • inform users of the residual risks due to any shortcomings of the protection measures adopted.

Reply:

3. The devices must achieve the performances intended by the manufacturer and be designed, manufactured and packaged in such a way that they are suitable for one or more of the functions referred to in Article 1(2)(a), as specified by the manufacturer.

Reply:

Medical Device Directive (93/42/EEC)
Annex I—Essential Requirements
Medical Device:_____
Page ___ of ___

4. The characteristics and performances referred to in Sections 1, 2 and 3 must not be adversely affected to such a degree that the clinical conditions and safety of the patients and, where applicable, of other persons are compromised during the lifetime of the device as indicated by the manufacturer, when the device is subjected to the stresses which can occur during normal conditions of use.

Reply:

5. The devices must be designed, manufactured and packed in such a way that their characteristics and performances during their intended use will not be adversely affected during transport and storage taking account of the instructions and information provided by the manufacturer.

Reply:

6. Any undesirable side-effect must constitute an acceptable risk when weighed against the performances intended.

Reply:

II. Requirements regarding design and construction

7. **Chemical, physical and biological properties**
7.1 The devices must be designed and manufactured in such a way as to guarantee the characteristics and performances referred to in Section I on the "General Requirements." Particular attention must be paid to:
   • the choice of materials used, particularly as regards toxicity and, where appropriate, flammability,

Medical Device Directive (93/42/EEC)
Annex I—Essential Requirements
Medical Device:_____
Page ____ of ____

- the compatibility between the materials used and biological tissues, cells and body fluids, taking account of the intended purpose of the device.

Reply:

7.2 The devices must be designed, manufactured and packed in such a way as to minimize the risk posed by contaminants and residues to the persons involved in the transport, storage and use of the devices and to the patients, taking account of the intended purpose of the product. Particular attention must be paid to the tissues exposed and to the duration and frequency of exposure.

Reply:

7.3 The devices must be designed and manufactured in such a way that they can be used safely with the materials, substances and gases with which they enter into contact during their normal use or during routine procedures; if the devices are intended to administer medicinal products, they must be designed and manufactured in such a way as to be compatible with the medicinal products concerned according to the provisions and restrictions governing these products and that their performance is maintained in accordance with the intended use.

Reply:

7.4 Where a device incorporates, as an integral part, a substance which, if used separately, may be considered to be a medicinal product, as defined in Article 1 of Directive 65/65/EEC, and which is liable to act upon the body with action ancillary to that of the device, the safety, quality and usefulness of the substance must be verified, taking ac-

Medical Device Directive (93/42/EEC)
Annex I—Essential Requirements
Medical Device:_____
Page ____ of ____

count of the intended purpose of the device, by analogy with the appropriate methods specified in Directive 75/318/EEC.

Reply:

7.5 The devices must be designed and manufactured in such a way as to reduce to a minimum the risks posed by substances leaking from the device.

Reply:

7.6 Devices must be designed and manufactured in such a way as to reduce, as much as possible, risks posed by the unintentional ingress of substances into the device taking into account the device and the nature of the environment in which it is intended to be used.

Reply:

8. Infection and microbial contamination
8.1 The devices and manufacturing processes must be designed in such a way as to eliminate or reduce as far as possible the risk of infection to the patient, user and third parties. The design must allow easy handling and, where necessary, minimize contamination of the device by the patient or vice versa during use.

Reply:

8.2 Tissues of animal origin must originate from animals that have been subjected to veterinary controls and surveillance adapted to the intended use of the tissues.
   • Notified bodies shall retain information on the geographical origin of the animals.

Medical Device Directive (93/42/EEC)
Annex I—Essential Requirements
Medical Device:_____
Page ____ of ____

- Processing, preservation, testing and handling of tissues, cells and substances of animal origin must be carried out so as to provide optimal security. In particular, safety with regard to viruses and other transferable agents must be addressed by implementation of validated methods of elimination or viral inactivation in the course of the manufacturing process.

Reply:

8.3 Devices delivered in a sterile state must be designed, manufactured and packed in a nonreusable pack and/or according to appropriate procedures to ensure that they are sterile when placed on the market and remain sterile, under the storage and transport conditions laid down, until the protective packaging is damaged or opened.

Reply:

8.4 Devices delivered in a sterile state must have been manufactured and sterilized by an appropriate, validated method.

Reply:

8.5 Devices intended to be sterilized must be manufactured in appropriately controlled (e.g., environmental) conditions.

Reply:

8.6 Packaging systems for nonsterile devices must keep the product without deterioration at the level of cleanliness stipulated and, if the devices are to be sterilized prior to use, minimize the risk of microbial

Medical Device Directive (93/42/EEC)
Annex I—Essential Requirements
Medical Device:_____
Page ____ of ____

---

contamination; the packaging system must be suitable taking account of the method of sterilization indicated by the manufacturer.

Reply:

8.7 The packaging and/or label of the device must distinguish between identical or similar products sold in both sterile and nonsterile condition.

Reply:

---

9. Construction and environmental properties
9.1 If the device is intended for use in combination with other devices or equipment, the whole combination, including the connection system, must be safe and must not impair the specified performances of the devices. Any restrictions on use must be indicated on the label or in the instructions for use.

Reply:

9.2 Devices must be designed and manufactured in such a way as to remove or minimize as far as is possible:
- the risk of injury, in connection with their physical features, including the volume/pressure ratio, dimensional and, where appropriate, ergonomic features,
- risks connected with reasonably foreseeable environmental conditions, such as magnetic fields, external electrical influences, electrostatic discharge, pressure, temperature or variations in pressure and acceleration,
- the risks of reciprocal interference with other devices normally used in the investigations or for the treatment given,

Medical Device Directive (93/42/EEC)
Annex I—Essential Requirements
Medical Device:_____
Page ___ of ___

- risks arising where maintenance or calibration are not possible (as with implants), from aging of materials used or loss of accuracy of any measuring or control mechanism.

Reply:

9.3 Devices must be designed and manufactured in such a way as to minimize the risks of fire or explosion during normal use and in single fault condition. Particular attention must be paid to devices whose intended use includes exposure to flammable substances or to substances which could cause combustion.

Reply:

---

10.   Devices with a measuring function
10.1 Devices with a measuring function must be designed and manufactured is such a way as to provide sufficient accuracy and stability within appropriate limits of accuracy and taking account of the intended purpose of the device. The limits of accuracy must be indicated by the manufacturer.

Reply:

10.2 The measurement, monitoring and display scale must be designed in line with ergonomic principles, taking account of the intended purpose of the device.

Reply:

Medical Device Directive (93/42/EEC)
Annex I—Essential Requirements
Medical Device:_____
Page ___ of ___

10.3. The measurements made by devices with a measuring function must be expressed in legal units conforming to the provisions of Council Directive 80/181/EEC.

Reply:

---

11. Protection against radiation
11.1 *General*
11.1.1 Devices shall be designed and manufactured in such a way that exposure of patients, users and other persons to radiation shall be reduced as far as possible compatible with the intended purpose, whilst not restricting the application of appropriate specified levels for therapeutic and diagnostic purposes.

Reply:

11.2 *Intended radiation*
11.2.1 Where devices are designed to emit hazardous levels of radiation necessary for a specific medical purpose, the benefit of which is considered to outweigh the risks inherent in the emission, it must be possible for the user to control the emissions. Such devices shall be designed and manufactured to ensure reproducibility and tolerance of relevant variable parameters.

Reply:

11.2.2 Where devices are intended to emit potentially hazardous, visible and/or invisible radiation, they must be fitted, where practicable, with visual displays and/or audible warnings of such emissions.

Reply:

Medical Device Directive (93/42/EEC)
Annex I—Essential Requirements
Medical Device:_____
Page ____ of ____

11.3   *Unintended radiation*
11.3.1 Devices shall be designed and manufactured in such a way that exposure of patients, users and other persons to the emission of unintended, stray or scattered radiation is reduced as far as possible.

Reply:

11.4   *Instructions*
11.4.1 The operating instructions for devices emitting radiation must give detailed information as to the nature of the emitted radiation, means of protecting the patient and the user and on ways of avoiding misuse and of eliminating the risks inherent in installation.

Reply:

11.5   *Ionizing radiation*
11.5.1 Devices intended to emit ionizing radiation must be designed and manufactured in such a way as to ensure that, where practicable, the quantity, geometry and quality of radiation emitted can be varied and controlled taking into account the intended use.

Reply:

11.5.2 Devices emitting ionizing radiation intended for diagnostic radiology shall be designed and manufactured in such a way as to achieve appropriate image and/or output quality for the intended medical purpose while minimizing radiation exposure of the patient and user.

Reply:

Medical Device Directive (93/42/EEC)
Annex I—Essential Requirements
Medical Device:_____
Page ___ of ___

11.5.3 Devices emitting ionizing radiation intended for therapeutic radiology shall be designed and manufactured in such a way as to enable reliable monitoring and control of the delivered dose, the beam type and energy and, where appropriate, the quality of radiation.

Reply:

---

12. Requirements for medical devices connected to or equipped with an energy source

12.1 Devices incorporating electronic programmable systems must be designed to ensure the repeatability, reliability and performance of these systems according to the intended use. In the event of a single fault condition (in the system), appropriate means should be adopted to eliminate or reduce as far as possible consequent risks.

Reply:

12.2 Devices where the safety of the patients depends on an internal power supply must be equipped with a means of determining the state of the power supply.

Reply:

12.3 Devices where the safety of the patients depends on an external power supply must include an alarm system to signal any power failure.

Reply:

Medical Device Directive (93/42/EEC)
Annex I—Essential Requirements
Medical Device: _____
Page ___ of ___

12.4 Devices intended to monitor one or more clinical parameters of a patient must be equipped with appropriate alarm systems to alert the user of situations which could lead to death or severe deterioration of the patient's state of health.
Reply:
12.5 Devices must be designed and manufactured in such a way as to minimize the risks of creating electromagnetic fields which could impair the operation of other devices or equipment in the usual environment.
Reply:
12.6 *Protection against electrical risks* Devices must be designed and manufactured in such a way as to avoid, as far as possible, the risk of accidental electric shocks during normal use and in single fault condition, provided the devices are installed correctly.
Reply:
12.7 *Protection against mechanical and thermal risks* 12.7.1 Devices must be designed and manufactured in such a way as to protect the patient and user against mechanical risks connected with, for example, resistance, stability and moving parts.
Reply:
12.7.2 Devices must be designed and manufactured in such a way as to reduce to the lowest possible level the risks arising from vibration generated by the devices, taking account of technical progress and

Medical Device Directive (93/42/EEC)
Annex I—Essential Requirements
Medical Device:_____
Page ____ of ____

| of the means available for limiting vibrations, particularly at source, unless the vibrations are part of the specified performance. |

Reply:

| 12.7.3 Devices must be designed and manufactured in such a way as to reduce to the lowest possible level the risks arising from the noise emitted, taking account of technical progress and of the means available to reduce noise, particularly at source, unless the noise emitted is part of the specified performance. |

Reply:

| 12.7.4 Terminals and connectors to the electricity, gas or hydraulic and pneumatic energy supplies which the user has to handle must be designed and constructed in such a way as to minimize all possible risks. |

Reply:

| 12.7.5 Accessible parts of the devices (excluding the parts or areas intended to supply heat or reach given temperatures) and their surroundings must not attain potentially dangerous temperatures under normal use. |

Reply:

| 12.8 *Protection against the risks posed to the patient by energy supplies or substances*
12.8.1 Devices for supplying the patient with energy or substances must be designed and constructed in such a way that the flow rate can be |

Medical Device Directive (93/42/EEC)
Annex I—Essential Requirements
Medical Device:_____
Page ____ of ____

set and maintained accurately enough to guarantee the safety of the patient and of the user.
Reply:
12.8.2 Devices must be fitted with the means of preventing and/or indicating any inadequacies in the flow rate which could pose a danger. • Devices must incorporate suitable means to prevent, as far as possible, the accidental release of dangerous levels of energy from an energy and/or substance source.
Reply:
12.9 The function of the controls and indicators must be clearly specified on the devices. • Where a device bears instructions required for its operation or indicates operating or adjustment parameters by means of a visual system, such information must be understandable to the user and, as appropriate, the patient.
Reply:
13.   Information supplied by the manufacturer 13.1 Each device must be accompanied by the information needed to use it safely and to identify the manufacturer, taking account of the training and knowledge of the potential users. • This information comprises the details on the label and the data in the instructions for use. • As far as practicable and appropriate, the information needed to use the device safely must be set out on the device itself and/or on the packaging for each unit or, where appropriate, on the sales packaging. If individual packaging of each unit is not practi-

Medical Device Directive (93/42/EEC)
Annex I—Essential Requirements
Medical Device:_____
Page ___ of ___

cable, the information must be set out in the leaflet supplied with one or more devices. • Instructions for use must be included in the packaging for every device. By way of exception, no such instructions for use are needed for devices in Class I or Class IIa if they can be used safely without any such instructions.
Reply:
13.2 Where appropriate, this information should take the form of symbols. Any symbol or identification color used must conform to the harmonized standards. In areas for which no standards exist, the symbols and colors must be described in the documentation supplied with the device.
Reply:
13.3 The label must bear the following particulars: (a) the name or trade name and address of the manufacturer. For devices imported into the Community, in view of their distribution in the Community, the label, or the outer packaging, or instructions for use, shall contain in addition the name and address of either the person responsible referred to in Article 14 (2) or of the authorized representative of the manufacturer established within the Community or of the importer established within the Community, as appropriate;
Reply:

Medical Device Directive (93/42/EEC)
Annex I—Essential Requirements
Medical Device:_____
Page ____ of ____

(b)	the details strictly necessary for the user to identify the device and the contents of the packaging;
Reply:	
(c)	where appropriate, the word "STERILE";
Reply:	
(d)	where appropriate, the batch code, preceded by the word "LOT," or the serial number;
Reply:	
(e)	where appropriate, an indication of the date by which the device should be used, in safety, expressed as the year and month;
Reply:	
(f)	where appropriate, an indication that the device is for single use;
Reply:	
(g)	if the device is custom-made, the words "custom-made device";
Reply:	
(h)	if the device is intended for clinical investigations, the words "exclusively for clinical investigations";
Reply:	

Medical Device Directive (93/42/EEC)
Annex I—Essential Requirements
Medical Device:_____
Page ____ **of** ____

(i)   any special storage and/or handling conditions;
Reply:
(j)   any special operating instructions;
Reply:
(k)   any warnings and/or precautions to take;
Reply:
(l)   year of manufacture for active devices other than those covered by (e). This indication may be included in the batch or serial number;
Reply:
(m)   where applicable, method of sterilization.
Reply:
13.4   If the intended purpose of the device is not obvious to the user, the manufacturer must clearly state it on the label and in the instructions for use.
Reply:
13.5   Wherever reasonable and practicable, the devices and detachable components must be identified, where appropriate in terms of

Medical Device Directive (93/42/EEC)
Annex I—Essential Requirements
Medical Device:_____
Page ____ of ____

batches, to allow all appropriate action to detect any potential risk posed by the devices and detachable components.
Reply:
13.6   Where appropriate, the instructions for use must contain the following particulars: (a)   the details referred to in Section 13.3, with the exception of points (d) and (e);
Reply:
(b)   the performances referred to in Section 3 and any undesirable side effects;
Reply:
(c)   if the device must be installed with or connected to other medical devices or equipment in order to operate as required for its intended purpose, sufficient details of its characteristics to identify the correct devices or equipment to use in order to obtain a safe combination;
Reply:
(d)   all the information needed to verify whether the device is properly installed and can operate correctly and safely, plus details of the nature and frequency of the maintenance and calibration needed to ensure that the devices operate properly and safely at all times;
Reply:

Medical Device Directive (93/42/EEC)
Annex I—Essential Requirements
Medical Device:_____
Page ____ of ____

(e)	where appropriate, information to avoid certain risks in connection with implantation of the device;
Reply:	
(f)	information regarding the risks of reciprocal interference posed by the presence of the device during specific investigations or treatment;
Reply:	
(g)	the necessary instructions in the event of damage to the sterile packaging and, where appropriate, details of appropriate methods of resterilization;
Reply:	
(h)	if the device is reusable, information on the appropriate processes to allow reuse, including cleaning, disinfection, packaging and, where appropriate, the method of sterilization of the device to be resterilized, and any restriction on the number of reuses. Where devices are supplied with the intention that they be sterilized before use, the instructions for cleaning and sterilization must be such that, if correctly followed, the device will still comply with the requirements of Section I;
Reply:	
(i)	details of any further treatment or handling needed before the device can be used (for example, sterilization, final assembly, etc.);
Reply:	

Medical Device Directive (93/42/EEC)
Annex I—Essential Requirements
Medical Device:_____
Page ____ of ____

(j)	in the case of devices emitting radiation for medical purposes, details of the nature, type, intensity and distribution of this radiation;
Reply:	
	The instructions for use must also include details allowing the medical staff to brief the patient on any contraindications and any precautions to be taken. These details should cover in particular:
(k)	precautions to be taken in the event of changes in the performance of the device;
Reply:	
(l)	precautions to be taken as regards exposure, in reasonably foreseeable environmental conditions, to magnetic fields, external electrical influences, electrostatic discharge, pressure or variations in pressure, acceleration, thermal ignition sources, etc.;
Reply:	
(m)	adequate information regarding medicinal product or products which the device in question is designed to administer, including any limitations in the choice of substances delivered;
Reply:	
(n)	precautions to be taken against special, unusual risks related to the disposal of the device;
Reply:	

Medical Device Directive (93/42/EEC)
Annex I—Essential Requirements
Medical Device:_____

Page ___ of ___

(o)   medicinal substances incorporated into the device as an integral part in accordance with Section 7.4;
Reply:
(p)   degree of accuracy claimed for devices with a measuring function.
Reply:
14.   Where conformity with the essential requirements must be based on clinical data, as in Section I (6), such data must be established in accordance with Annex X.
Reply:

Chapter 7

Conformity Assessment Routes
Overview

One of the more complex activities facing a medical device manufacturer seeking to comply with MDD requirements entails selecting a conformity assessment route. Manufacturers are given a choice of paths by which they can meet the directive's requirements; the class attributed to the product will determine the route they must follow. The conformity procedures basically address two stages: design and manufacture.

For design, manufacturers must provide objective evidence of how the device meets essential requirements. This technical information should be held within a technical file, or design dossier. For manufacture, a documented quality system must be in place to ensure that the devices continue to comply with essential requirements and are consistent with the information in the technical file.

Annexes II, III, IV, V, VI, VII and VIII identify conformity assessment routes. Most of these annexes require the manufacturer's quality system to be assessed and comply with the applicable EN 46000 series standard. Those assessments must be conducted by a notified body (or through an agreement with another organization) authorized to perform MDD assessments.

Because device classification determines the appropriate conformity assessment route, this important step in the overall process must be made on an informed basis. Manufacturers would be wise to seek the counsel of a notified body to assist them in this activity.

The modular approach
For the reader who has reviewed the MDD with its general lack of clarity, it should come as no surprise that the various annexes in the directive have little consistency with the various conformity assessment modules identified in Directive 93/465/EEC (CE Conformity Marking). In a sense, the two can be analyzed to show that Module II, for example, is similar to an Annex II (full quality assurance system) method of meeting

the directive's requirements and allowing use of the CE Mark. To make matters worse, more than one module can be applied to a product or service.

Chapter 4 reviews and explains the annexes for conformity assessment; this chapter will review the various modules and the modular approach of conformity assessment. The modular approach separates conformity assessments procedures into a number of operations (modules) that differ with respect to the product's state of development, the assessment type and the party performing the assessment; the modules can then be combined to form a total process. This approach permits an easier evaluation of the processes and procedures. The modular approach evaluates two distinct process stages: design and production. For example, Module C can be used with Module B; modules D, E and F are generally combined with Module B, but in special cases they may be used on their own. The complexity can be very disconcerting.

However, not all modules are authorized for use with the MDD; this may result in less frustration.

Module A: Internal Production Control

This module addresses both the design and production stages of the process. The basic requirements allow the manufacturer to declare that the products satisfy the requirements of the applicable directive. The manufacturer or authorized representative is responsible for retaining the appropriate documentation and technical files as objective evidence of compliance with the directive and must make those documents available to the notified body and/or competent authority. The manufacturer or authorized representative is then permitted to apply the CE Mark to the applicable products and prepare (and retain) the written declaration of conformity.

With respect to the MDD, manufacturers must meet all applicable requirements, particularly those in Annex I. This module provides another way for manufacturers of Class I medical devices to get the CE Mark on their products and is virtually identical to an Annex VII conformity assessment route.

Module B: EC Type-Examination

This module applies only to the design phase; manufacturers must use a complementary production module in conjunction with Module B.

Under this methodology, the notified body must declare (*ascertain and attest,* using the directive's language) that a representative sample of the product meets the applicable requirements that apply to the product. The notified body must evaluate the manufacturer's technical documentation and perform those tests and inspections necessary to demonstrate product conformity to the provisions of the MDD, for example. Once the notified body completes all required activities and the product is found to be in compliance, it issues an EC type-examination certificate to the manufacturer; if the manufacturer is denied an EC type certificate, the notified body must provide a detailed explanation and justification for such denial. An appeals process must be made available to the manufacturer.

At this time, the CE Mark is not affixed to the product because only the design phase has been assessed. Module B is a close equivalent to the requirements in Annex III of the MDD, as they apply to the design stage.

As stated earlier, once manufacturers elect to use Module B for the product's design phase, they must also select a supporting production module: C, D, E or F.

Module C: Conformity to Type

Module C basically is a declaration of conformity by the manufacturer for the "marketable" (i.e., commercial product in the production phase) device to support an EC type-examination by the notified body. Having satisfactorily achieved Module B, the manufacturer or authorized representative declares that the products satisfy the applicable directive's requirements. The manufacturer or authorized representative is responsible for retaining the appropriate documentation and technical files as objective evidence of compliance with the directive and must supply those documents to the notified body and/or competent authority. The manufacturer or authorized representative is then permitted to apply the CE Mark to the products and prepare (and retain) the written declaration of conformity.

The manufacturer must meet all applicable MDD requirements, particularly those in Annex I. This module is similar to an Annex III/Annex VII approach for conformity assessment (because it must be used in conjunction with Module B).

Module D: Production Quality Assurance

Manufacturers use Module D when operating an approved quality system (e.g., ISO 9002 and/or EN 46002) for production, final inspection and testing that has been assessed by a notified body to support an EC type-examination by the notified body. The manufacturer is also subject to periodic surveillance assessments by the notified body.

Used for medical devices, Module D combines the requirements of Annex III and Annex V to achieve conformity assessment. All applicable MDD requirements, both for the essential requirements in Annex I and the conformity assessment route specified in Annex V, must be met before the manufacturer or authorized representative can affix the CE Mark to the medical device.

Module E: Product Quality Assurance

Module E is used when a manufacturer operates an approved quality system (e.g., ISO 9001/ISO 9002 and/or EN 46001/EN 46002) for final inspection and testing that has been assessed by a notified body to support an EC type-examination by the notified body. The manufacturer is also subject to periodic surveillance assessments by the notified body.

Used for medical devices, Module E combines the requirements of Annex III and Annex VI to achieve conformity assessment. All applicable MDD requirements, both for the essential requirements in Annex I and the conformity assessment route specified in Annex VI, must be met before the manufacturer or authorized representative can affix the CE Mark to the medical device.

Module F: Product Verification

With Module F, a notified body declares that the product conforms with the technical documentation or with the type as described in the EC type-examination certificate to support an EC type-examination by the notified body. In either case, products must satisfy the MDD requirements that apply to them.

Manufacturers may elect to use statistical verification as opposed to 100-percent verification provided they take all necessary steps to ensure homogeneity among lots and within each lot. Random samples must then be selected. After meeting all requirements, the manufacturer or authorized representative then may apply the CE Mark to the products and prepare (and retain) the written declaration of conformity.

Used for medical devices, Module F combines the requirements of Annex III and Annex IV to achieve conformity assessment. All applicable MDD requirements, both for the essential requirements in Annex I and the conformity assessment route specified in Annex IV, must be met before the manufacturer or authorized representative can affix the CE Mark to the medical device.

Module G: Unit Verification

Module G relates to both the design and production phases of the process and is normally used for unit production or for small lots/batches. The notified body declares that individual products comply with the applicable directive requirements. In the case of this module, the notified body must affix the CE Mark to the product and prepare the declaration of conformity.

Module G is *not* authorized for use with medical devices.

Module H: Full Quality Assurance

Module H relates to both the design and production stages of a manufacturer's process. The manufacturer operates an approved quality system (e.g., ISO 9001 and/or EN 46001) for design, production, final inspection and testing that has been assessed by a notified body. The manufacturer is also subject to periodic surveillance assessments by the notified body.

With respect to the MDD, the manufacturer must meet all applicable deadline requirements, particularly those in Annex I. This module is virtually identical to an Annex II conformity assessment route.

The following table depicts the procedures for using conformity assessment modules and how they relate to the MDD annexes:

Table 7.1: Conformity Assessment Modules

Module	Phase	MDD Annex
A	Design, production	VII
B	Design	III
C*	Production	VII (with III)
D*	Production	V (with III)
E*	Production	VI (with III)
F*	Production	IV (with III)
G	Design, production	Not permitted
H	Design, production	II

*Must be used in conjunction with Module B

Chapter 8

Use of the CE Mark
Identifying the product

The CE Mark (CE marking) symbolizes conformity with all requirements and obligations incumbent on the manufacturer of the medical device relative to the product. The CE Mark affixed to medical devices symbolizes the fact that the individual who has affixed or who is responsible for affixing the CE Mark has verified that the product conforms to all European Union harmonization requirements that apply to the device and that the device has been assessed for compliance to the appropriate conformity assessment procedures. Where devices are subject to additional directives concerning other aspects and that also provide for affixing the CE Mark, manufacturers also must comply with these requirements.

CE marking requirements

1. The CE Mark must consist of the initials "CE," taking the following form:

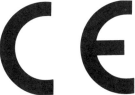

If the marking is reduced or enlarged, the manufacturer must use the given proportions.

2. For medical devices, the various CE Mark components must have substantially the same vertical dimension, which may not be less than 5 mm. The minimum dimension may be waived for small devices.

3. The CE Mark must be affixed to the product or to its data plate. Where it is not possible or warranted due to the product's nature, the CE Mark must be affixed to the packaging (if any) and to any accompanying documents.

4. The CE Mark must be affixed visibly, legibly and indelibly.

5. The CE Mark must be affixed at the end of the production control phase and must be followed by the notified body's identification number.

6. The CE Mark and the notified body's identification number *may* be followed by a pictogram or other mark indicating, for example, the category of use.

7. The affixing of any other mark, sign or indication that may potentially deceive third parties as to the meaning and form of the CE Mark is prohibited.

8. A medical device may bear different marks (e.g., indicating conformity with national or European standards or additional directives) provided that such marks do not cause confusion with the CE Mark.

9. The CE Mark must be affixed by the manufacturer or authorized representative established within the European Union.

10. Member states are authorized to take all required steps to exclude any possibility of confusion and to prevent abuse of the CE Mark.

Chapter 9

Notified Bodies
Verification of compliance

The MDD defines the criteria an organization must meet to be designated a notified body. A notified body is defined as "a government-sanctioned organization that can register and/or certify a quality system or product and determine that the system or product meets the European Union requirements." The notified body should not be confused with a registrar ("an accredited third party that evaluates an organization's quality system to verify compliance with the applicable requirements") or a competent authority ("the regulatory body within a member state that is charged with ensuring that the provisions of the MDD are correctly implemented.") As an example, for medical devices within the United Kingdom, the competent authority is the Secretary of State for Health acting through the Medical Devices Agency.

A notified body must comply with seven basic requirements, as follows:

1. The notified body, its management, and assessment and verification staff cannot be the designer, manufacturer, supplier, installer, authorized representative or user of the devices that they inspect. They cannot be directly involved with the design, manufacture, marketing or maintenance of the device or represent the parties involved with those activities.

In other words, the notified body must be independent of the activities that they assess.

2. The notified body and its staff must perform its assessment and verification activities with professional integrity. Personnel must be competent in the field of medical devices and must be free from any pressures and inducements (particularly financial) that may influence their judgment or the results of the activities that they perform.

If the notified body subcontracts specific tasks, it must ensure that the subcontractor meets the same provisions and criteria that the notified body must meet.

In other words, the notified body must be honest and ethical.

3. The notified body must be able to perform all activities in annexes II through VI. It must have the necessary personnel, facilities and equipment needed to properly perform the technical and administrative tasks entailed in assessment and verification activities.

In other words, the notified body must have appropriate resources to perform the activities required by the MDD.

4. The notified body must have suitable training covering all assessment and verification activities for which it has been designated by the competent authority, satisfactory knowledge and experience in the products and standards and regulations applicable for medical devices, and the ability to prepare and issue the necessary certificates, records and reports to demonstrate that the activities have been performed.

In other words, the notified body must have the appropriate industry background, experience and expertise, and a system to verify its activities.

5. The notified body must be impartial, and fees cannot depend on the results of inspections or the number of inspections performed.

In other words, the notified body must be financially independent.

6. The notified body must carry adequate insurance.

In other words, the notified body must take precautions against potential liability in a litigious society.

7. Personnel of the notified body are required to maintain professional secrecy and confidentiality with respect to *all* information obtained during the course of their duties pursuant to the MDD.

In other words, nothing that the notified body sees, hears or reads goes anywhere beyond the organization being assessed and its own staff.

Chapter 10

Supporting Requirements
Standards and regulations

Previous mention has been made about the Annex II (or Module H) method of conformity assessment to the MDD. For those organizations that have a registered quality system, the full quality assurance system methodology of CE marking its products makes a great deal of administrative and economic sense. However, this method requires an organization to meet all applicable regulatory requirements and to be registered to the applicable ISO 9000 and EN 46000 standards.

For those not familiar with the EN 46000 or ISO 13485 documents, they are the additional requirements to ISO 9001:1994 that apply to medical devices. The EN 46000 standards are European Norms that apply to European Union member states (and those countries that want to export into the European Union); ISO 13485 is an international standard under the auspices of the International Organization for Standardization that will eventually replace EN 46001. These two documents will be discussed in more detail later in this chapter.

In the United States, medical device manufacturers must comply with a myriad of regulatory requirements. These include the new Quality System Regulation (21 CFR 820, formally known as the Medical Device Good Manufacturing Practices), the Medical Device Reporting legislation (21 CFR 803), Guidelines on the Principles of Process Validation, and the Safe Medical Devices Act of 1990.

For the purposes of this discussion, it will be assumed that the reader is familiar with the regulatory requirements, including the Quality System Regulation that has recently been enacted (June 1, 1997, with the exception of those for design control, which become effective June 1, 1998.)

EN 46001 provides particular requirements for medical device manufacturers that are more specific than ISO 9001's general requirements. Because compliance with EN 46001 is required for a variety of conformity assessment routes, the reader must understand that:

• It is *not* the same as ISO 9001.

- It is *not* the same as the MDD.
- It is *not* the same as the Good Manufacturing Practices/Quality System Regulation.
- It includes the additional requirements for medical devices over and above the requirements of an ISO 9001-registered system.
- The current document is the August 1996 revision of the standard.

The author has assessed organizations that have made erroneous hypotheses which have resulted in a delay in CE marking their medical devices. To paraphrase a popular proverb, "Ignorance of the requirements is no excuse." Therefore, EN 46001:1996 defines the following additional requirements, which organizations should incorporate into their documented quality system.

For all medical devices

4.2—Quality System. The supplier shall establish and document the specified requirements.

The supplier must establish and maintain a file containing documents defining the product specifications, including complete manufacturing and quality assurance specifications for each type/model of medical device, or referring to the location of this information.

4.4—Design Control. The supplier shall identify requirements that are related to the safety of the medical device and shall include such requirements as design input data.

The supplier must document and maintain records of all design verification activities, including those involving clinical investigation.

4.5—Document and Data Control. The supplier shall define the period for which at least one copy of an obsolete document shall be retained. This period shall ensure that specifications to which medical devices have been manufactured are available for at least the lifetime of the medical device, as defined by the supplier.

4.6—Purchasing. To the extent required by the particular traceability requirements, the supplier shall retain copies of relevant purchasing documents.

4.8—Product Identification and Traceability. The supplier shall establish and maintain procedures to ensure that medical devices received for refurbishing are identified and distinguished at all times from normal production.

The supplier must establish, document and maintain traceability procedures. The procedures must define the extent of traceability and facilitate corrective action.

4.9—Process Control.

• *Personnel.* The supplier must establish, document and maintain requirements for health, cleanliness and clothing of personnel if contact between such personnel and product or environment could adversely affect product quality.

• *Environmental Control in Manufacture.* For medical devices that are supplied sterile *or* that are supplied nonsterile and intended for sterilization before use *or* where the microbiological and/or particulate cleanliness or other environmental conditions are of significance in their use *or* where the environmental conditions are of significance in their manufacture, the supplier must establish and document requirements for the environment to which the product is exposed. If appropriate, the environmental conditions must be controlled and/or monitored.

• *Cleanliness of Product.* The supplier must establish, document and maintain requirements for cleanliness of product if product is cleaned by the supplier prior to sterilization and/or its use *or* product is supplied nonsterile to be subjected to a cleaning process prior to sterilization and/or its use *or* product is supplied to be used nonsterile and its cleanliness is of significance in use *or* process agents are to be removed from product during manufacture. If appropriate, product cleaned prior to sterilization and/or use need not be subject to the preceding personnel or environmental control requirements.

• *Maintenance.* The supplier must establish and document requirements for maintenance activities when such activities may affect product quality. Records of such maintenance shall be maintained.

• *Installation.* If appropriate, the supplier must establish and document both instructions and acceptance criteria for installing and checking the medical device. Records of installation and checking performed by the supplier or authorized representative must be retained. If the contract allows installation other than by the supplier or authorized representative, the supplier must provide the purchaser with written instructions for installation and checking.

• *Special Processes.* The supplier must ensure that the quality records of special processes identify the work instruction used, the date that the special process was performed and the identity of the operator of the special process.

4.13—Control of Nonconforming Product. The supplier shall ensure that nonconforming product is accepted by concession (waiver) only if regulatory requirements are met. The identity of the person authorizing the concession shall be recorded.

If product needs to be reworked, the supplier must document the rework in a work instruction that has undergone the same authorization and approval procedure as the original work instruction.

4.14—Corrective and Preventive Action. The supplier shall establish and maintain a documented feedback system to provide early warning of quality problems and for input into the corrective action system. If EN 46001:1996 is used for compliance with regulatory requirements that require post-marketing surveillance, the surveillance shall form part of the feedback system.

All feedback information, including reported customer complaints and returned product, must be documented, investigated, interpreted, collated and communicated in accordance with defined procedures by a designated person. If any customer complaint is not followed by corrective action, the reason must be recorded.

The supplier must maintain records of all complaint investigations. When the investigation determines that the activities at remote premises played a part in the complaint, a copy of the report must be sent to those premises. If EN 46001:1996 is used for compliance with regulatory requirements, the supplier must establish, document and maintain procedures to notify the regulatory authority of those incidents that meet the reporting criteria.

The supplier must establish, document and maintain procedures for the issue of advisory notices and the recall of medical devices. These procedures must be capable of being implemented at any time.

4.15—Handling, Storage, Packaging, Preservation and Delivery. The supplier shall establish and maintain documented procedures for the control of product with a limited shelf life or requiring special storage conditions. Such special storage conditions shall be controlled and recorded.

If appropriate, special provisions must be made for the handling of used product in order to prevent contamination of other product, the manufacturing environment or personnel.

4.16—Control of Quality Records. The supplier shall retain the quality records for a period of time at least equivalent to the lifetime of the medical device defined by the supplier, but not less than two years from the date of shipment from the supplier.

The supplier must establish and maintain a record for each batch of medical devices that provides traceability to the extent required by element 4.8 and identifies the quantity manufactured and quantity released for distribution. The batch record must be verified and authorized.

4.18—Training. The supplier shall ensure that all personnel who are required to work under special environmental conditions or who perform special processes or functions are appropriately trained or supervised by a trained person.

4.20—Statistical Techniques. The supplier shall establish and maintain procedures to ensure that sampling methods are regularly reviewed in the light of the occurrence of nonconforming product, quality audit reports, feedback information and other appropriate considerations.

For sterile medical devices

In addition to the requirements listed above for all medical devices, the following supplementary provisions apply:

4.9—Process Control. The supplier shall subject the medical devices to a validated sterilization process and record all the control parameters of the sterilization process.

4.15—Handling, Storage, Packaging, Preservation and Delivery. The supplier shall establish and maintain procedures to ensure that the medical device is presented in a container that maintains the medical device's sterility, except for those medical devices for which only the inner surfaces are sterile and the medical device is such that the sterility of the inner surfaces is maintained.

The supplier must establish and maintain procedures to ensure that the medical device can be presented in an aseptic manner, if its use so requires.

The supplier must establish and maintain procedures to ensure that the package, or medical device if only the inner surface is sterile, clearly reveals that it has been opened.

For active implantable medical devices

In addition to the requirements listed above for all medical devices, the following supplementary provisions apply:

4.8—Product Identification and Traceability. The extent of traceability shall include all components and materials used, and records of the environmental conditions, when these could cause the medical device not to satisfy its specified requirements.

4.10—Inspection and Testing. The supplier shall record the identity of personnel performing any inspection or testing.

4.15—Handling, Storage, Packaging, Preservation and Delivery. The supplier shall record the identity of persons who perform the final labeling operation.

The supplier must ensure that the name and address of the shipping package consignee is included in the quality records.

The supplier must require that any authorized representative maintain records of medical device distribution and that such records are available for inspection.

For implantable medical devices

In addition to the requirements listed above for all medical devices, the following supplementary provisions apply:

4.8—Product Identification and Traceability. The extent of traceability shall include all components and materials used, and records of the environmental conditions, when these could cause the medical device not to satisfy its specified requirements.

4.10—Inspection and Testing. The supplier shall record the identity of personnel performing any inspection or testing.

4.15—Handling, Storage, Packaging, Preservation and Delivery. The supplier shall record the identity of persons who perform the final labeling operation.

The supplier must ensure that the name and address of the shipping package consignee is included in the quality records.

The supplier must require that any authorized representative maintain records of medical device distribution and that such records are available for inspection.

A review of these requirements will result in the conclusion that compliance with federal regulatory requirements would generally result in compliance with EN 46001.

Chapter 11

Summary

At this point, the reader should have a fairly broad understanding of the CE Mark and the associated requirements for medical devices. While the language and grammar used in the MDD leave something to be desired, the document's intent is clear and of great value. There are few, if any, provisions in the directive that medical device manufacturers located in the United States should not already have implemented in the quest to keep the Food and Drug Administration from enacting sanctions against them.

Chapter 1 reviewed the European Union and the basis for enacting the various directives—primarily to ensure quality and safety in product lines that it felt were warranted. Chapter 2 provided an overview of the MDD and the document's contents.

Chapters 3, 4 and 6 provided detailed analyses of the articles and annexes comprising the MDD and attempted to clarify the confusing structure and language used.

Chapter 5 explained how devices are classified using the definitions provided in the directive, and Chapter 7 furnished an alternative scheme, the modular approach, for conformity assessment and CE marking of medical devices. Once manufacturers meet all applicable requirements and can affix the CE Mark to their products, Chapter 8 defines the stipulations for that activity. Chapter 9 explained the rules and regulations under which notified bodies must perform.

Chapter 10 identified the other various standards and regulations which apply to an organization that wishes to meet the MDD requirements through the full quality assurance system conformity assessment route.

If this book were any longer and detailed, it would not accomplish its intended purpose. It has summarized those areas needing interpretation and clarification without creating a massive tome of valueless trivia. Armed with this book, the applicable quality system standards and the pertinent regulations, the reader should possess the relevant information needed to understand and, hopefully, comply with the directive's requirements.

Appendix 1

Examples of Other European Union Directives

Following is a listing of other directives promulgated by the European Union. Those identified with an asterisk (*) may also apply to medical device manufacturers.

*Active Implantable Medical Devices
Appliances
Articles of Precious Metals (Proposal)
Construction Products
*Cosmetic Products
*Electromagnetic Compatibility
*Electromedical Equipment
Explosives for Civil Use
*Good Laboratory Practices
*Good Manufacturing Practices
*Human Medicinal Products
*In-Vitro Diagnostics (Proposal)
Lifts
Low Voltage
Machinery Safety
Marine Equipment (Proposal)
*Measuring Equipment (Proposal)
*Medical Device
*Module of Conformity Assessment
New Hot Water Boilers
Personal Protective Equipment
Pleasure Crafts
Potential Explosive Atmospheres
Pressure Vessels
*Risk Assessment
Telecommunications Terminal Equipment
Toys

Appendix 2

Examples of Nonmedical Devices

The following product examples are *not* considered to be medical devices unless a medical claim is being made by the manufacturer of the device:

Products intended for toiletry or cosmetic purposes
- Toothbrushes, dental sticks, dental floss, unmedicated dental chewing gums
- Baby diapers, mattress protectors, hygienic tampons or napkins
- Contact lenses without corrective function intended to provide another eye color
- Instruments for tattooing
- Deodorants for use with devices
- Wigs

Personal protective equipment
- Self-rescue apparatus
- Mouthguards
- Ionizing radiation protective clothing
- Eye protecting visors
- Protective gloves

Other equipment
- Acoustic signals at traffic lights
- Breathalyzers, other blood or air alcohol measuring devices
- Nonsterile home, occupational, recreational protective or safety apparel
- Nonprescription sunglasses
- Consumer products aimed at comfort products for sport or leisure

Appendix 3

Examples of Class I Medical Devices

The following product examples are considered to be Class I medical devices:

Administrative Devices
- Measuring cups, spoons, droppers
- Inhalation devices
- Solution and irrigation sets
- Hypodermic and oral syringes
- Dispensers
- Sensitivity testing devices
- Nonactive autoinjector devices

Dental Devices
- Dental lights
- Dental diagnostic fiber optic handpieces
- Dental instruments, reusable, nonpowered
- Dental prophylaxis paste (nonfluoride)
- Handheld dental mirrors
- Impression materials
- Orthodontic materials (extra-oral parts only)
- Retraction cords, dental wedges, rubber dams, matrix bands
- Articulating paper
- Dental waxes
- Dental unit accessories
- Artificial teeth
- Base materials
- Dental mouthwash tablets (nonmedicated)

Diagnostic Devices
- Conductive gels
- Noninvasive electrodes and accessories

- Peak flow meters
- Sphygmomanometers
- Stethoscopes
- Clinical thermometers
- Examination and procedure gloves
- Blood sampling devices (reusable)
- Endoscopes, endoscopic instruments and accessories
- Image storage and retrieval systems
- Laryngoscopes, otoscopes and accessories
- X-ray cassettes

Dressings and Bandages
- Bandages
- Cotton, wool, gauze, nonwoven
- Adhesive plasters and tapes
- Eye occlusion plasters and shields
- Chiropody dressings and pads

Equipment and Furnishings (other than stated elsewhere)
- Allergen-resistant bedding
- Examination couches
- Hospital beds
- Patient hoists
- Pressure relief devices and accessories
- Treatment chairs
- Hospital trolleys
- Traction devices
- Medical examination luminaries
- Rehabilitation equipment
- Splints and collars

Ophthalmic Devices
- Ophthalmic examination lamps
- Fundas cameras, keratometers, slit lamp microscopes
- Low vision aids
- Operating room microscopes
- Ophthalmoscopes and retinoscopes
- Spectacle lenses
- Spectacle frames

- Ready-made spectacles (nonprescription)
- Sight-testing devices

Orthopedics and Prosthetics
- Orthopedic footwear (other than custom-made)
- Orthotics (lower and upper limb, spinal, abdominal, neck, head)
- Trusses
- Compression hosiery and garments
- External limb prostheses (other than custom-made)
- Stump socks
- Orthopedic casting and support products

Surgical Devices (other than those stated elsewhere)
- Umbilical clamps
- Esophageal and rectal tubes
- Enema devices
- Incision drapes and operating room clothing
- Surgical instruments (reusable, nonpowered)
- Pre-operative devices (e.g., razors, marker pens)
- Airway devices and accessories
- Noninvasive drainage devices
- Surgical instrument accessories
- Sterilization packaging

Mobility Aids
- Crutches and walking sticks
- Walking frames and standing frames
- Rollators and mobilators
- Wheelchairs (nonpowered)
- Wheelchairs (powered)
- For the visually impaired

Waste-Collection Devices
- Ostomy collection devices and accessories
- Incontinence pads and accessories
- Urinary bags and accessories
- Noninvasive tubing
- Penile sheaths
- Urinary catheters (intermittent)

Appendix 4

Examples of Custom-Made Devices

The following examples of products are considered custom-made if they are manufactured in accordance with a professional's written prescription for the sole use of a particular patient and are not adapted from mass-produced items.

- Dental appliances and prostheses
- Hearing aid inserts
- Prescribed orthopedic footwear
- Artificial eyes
- External orthotics and prosthetics (made direct from casts)
- Joint replacement implants
- Maxillo-facial devices

Appendix 5

Classification Routes: Noninvasive Chart

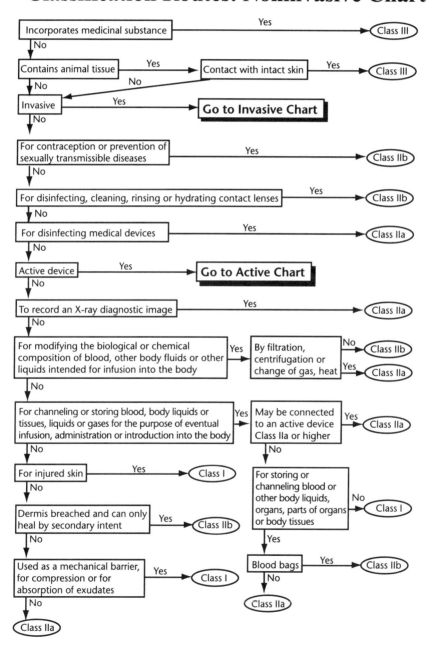

Appendix 6

Classification Routes: Invasive Chart

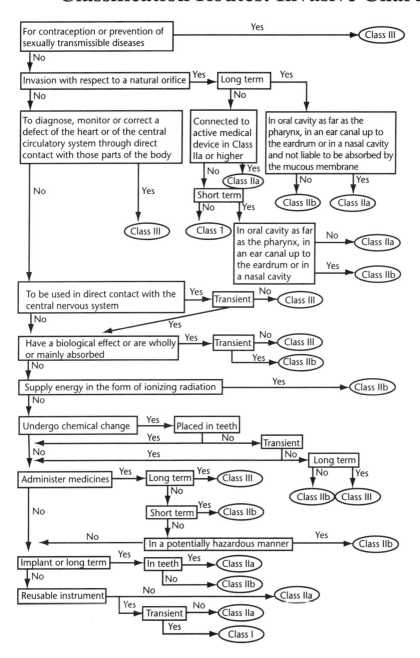

Appendix 7

Classification Routes: Active Chart

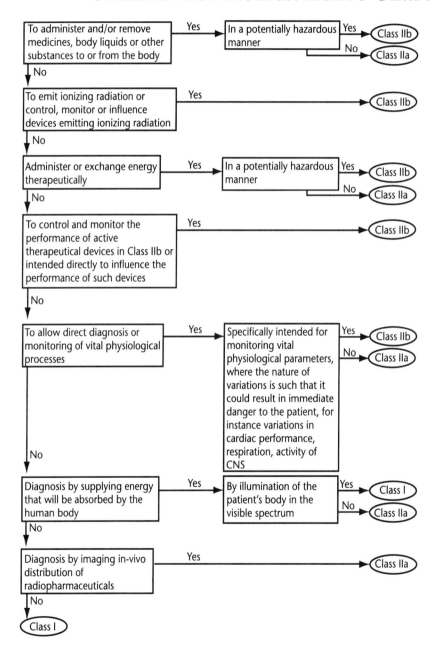

Appendix 8

Declaration of Conformity
Application of Council Directive 93/42/EEC

Manufacturer's Name: _____

Manufacturer's Address: _____

_____

_____

Name of Equipment: _____

Type No., Model No.
or Reference No.: _____

Serial Number(s): _____

Year of Manufacture: _____

I, the undersigned, hereby declare that the
equipment specified above conforms
to Directive 93/42/EEC

Place: _____

Name: _____

Signature: _____

Position: _____

Glossary

Accessory

An article that, while not being a device, is intended specifically by its manufacturer to be used together with a device to enable it to be used in accordance with the use of the device intended by the manufacturer of the device.

Accredited/Accreditation

The procedure by which an authoritative body (e.g., a notified body) gives formal recognition that a body or person (e.g., a registrar) is competent to perform specific tasks and activities.

Active Device for Diagnosis

Any active medical device, whether used alone or in combination with other medical devices, to supply information for detecting, diagnosing, monitoring or treating physiological conditions, states of health, illnesses or congenital deformities.

Active Implantable Medical Device

Any active medical device intended to be totally or partially introduced, surgically or medically, into the human body or by medical intervention into a natural orifice, and that is intended to remain after the procedure.

Active Medical Device

Any medical device relying for its functioning on a source of electrical energy or any source of power other than that directly generated by the human body or by gravity. Medical devices intended to transmit energy, substances or other elements between an active medical device and the patient without significant change are not considered to be active medical devices.

Active Therapeutic Device

Any active medical device, whether used alone or in combination with other medical devices, to support, modify, replace or restore biological functions or structures with a view to treatment or alleviation of an illness, injury or handicap.

Authorized Representative

A person or organization appointed by a medical device manufacturer to whom precise tasks and duties are delegated. All authorized representatives must be established (i.e., have a registered business) in the European Union.

Body Orifice

Any natural opening in the body, as well as the external surface of the eyeball, or any permanent artificial opening (such as a stoma).

CE Mark/CE Marking

A blanket mark stating that a product meets all of the European Union regulatory requirements for that specific product/product line. The CE Mark must appear in a visible, legible and indelible form on the device or its sterile pack, where practical and appropriate, and on any instructions for use in sales packaging, where appropriate.

CEN

Committee for European Norms, also referred to as the European Commission for Standardization. CEN develops nonelectrical standards for determining product compliance.

CENELEC

European Commission for Electrotechnical Standardization. CENELEC develops electrical standards for product compliance.

Central Circulatory System

For purposes of the MDD, the central circulatory system includes the pulmonary arteries, ascending aorta, coronary arteries, carotid arteries, cerebral arteries, brachycephalicus truck, vena cava and pulmonary veins.

Central Nervous System

For purposes of the MDD, the central nervous system includes the brain, meninges and spinal cord.

Certified/Certification

A procedure by which a third party provides written assurance that a product or service conforms to requirements. Also, the process by which third-party lead assessors/assessors are judged to be competent to perform assessments.

Commission
The arm of the European Union whose primary function is to implement the directives and regulations.

Competent Authority
The regulatory body within a member state that is charged with ensuring that the MDD provisions are correctly implemented. As an example, for medical devices within the United Kingdom, the competent authority is the Secretary of State for Health acting through the Medical Devices Agency.

Council
The European Union arm whose primary function is to write directives and regulations.

Custom-Made Device
Any device specifically made in accordance with a duly qualified medical practitioner's written prescription that gives, under his or her responsibility, specific design characteristics and is intended for the sole use of a particular patient.

Declaration of Conformity
The procedure whereby the manufacturer or authorized representative prepares the required technical documentation, implements corrective action and vigilance procedures, and declares that the products meet the essential requirements defined in MDD Annex I.

Device Intended for Clinical Investigation
Any device intended for use by a duly qualified medical practitioner when conducting investigations.

Directive
A rule or regulation enacted by the European Union that is binding on the member states to which they apply.

EN 45000
A series of guidelines that defines a level of performance for laboratories.

EN 46000
A series of guidelines that provides additional requirements for applying the ISO 9000 series of standards to medical devices.

European Free Trade Association (EFTA)
Consists of Iceland, Liechtenstein and Norway. The European Community merged with EFTA on January 1, 1994, to form the European Economic Area.

European Union (EU)
Consists of Austria, Belgium, Denmark, Finland, France, Germany, Greece, Ireland, Italy, Luxembourg, the Netherlands, Portugal, Spain, Sweden and the United Kingdom.

Harmonized/Harmonized Standard
A technical specification that has been adopted by either CEN or CENELEC and states the procedure for supplying information regarding technical standards and regulations.

Implantable Device
Any device intended to be totally introduced into the human body or to replace an epithelial surface or the surface of the eye by surgical intervention and that is intended to remain in place after the procedure.

Intended Purpose
The use for which the medical device is intended according to the data supplied by the manufacturer on the labeling, instructions and/or promotional materials.

International Electrotechnical Commission (IEC)
An organization that establishes internationally recognized and accepted standards in the fields of electrical and electronic engineering.

International Organization for Standardization (ISO)
An international organization comprised of the national standards bodies of more than 100 countries that promotes the development of standardiza-

tion and related world activities with a view to facilitating international exchange of goods and services.

Invasive Device
A device that, in whole or in part, penetrates inside the body, either through a body orifice or through the surface of the body.

In-Vitro Diagnostic
Any device that is a reagent, reagent product, kit, instrument, equipment or system, whether used alone or in combination, intended by the manufacturer to be used *in vitro* for examining samples derived from the human body with a view to providing information on the physiological state of health, disease or congenital abnormality.

ISO 9000
A broad-based, generic series of documents that, when followed, assures that customers receive reliable and consistent quality products and services.

ISO 13485
An international standard that will replace the EN 46000 guidelines as the documents that provide additional requirements for applying the ISO 9000 series of standards to medical devices.

Long-Term Device
A device normally intended for continuous use for more than 30 days.

Manufacturer
The natural or legal person with responsibility for the design, manufacture, packaging and labeling of a device before it is placed on the market under his or her own name, regardless of whether these operations are performed by that person or by another on his or her behalf.

Medical Device
Any instrument, apparatus, appliance, material or other article, whether used alone or in combination, including the software necessary for its proper application, intended by the manufacturer to be used for human beings for the purposes of:
• Diagnosis, prevention, monitoring, treatment or alleviation of disease
• Diagnosis, monitoring, treatment or alleviation of or compensation for

an injury or handicap
• Investigation, replacement or modification of the anatomy or of a physiological process
• Control of conception

and which does not achieve its principal intended action in or on the human body by pharmacological, immunological or metabolic means, but which may be assisted in its function by such means.

Medicinal Product
A product that achieves its principal action by pharmacological, immunological or metabolic means.

Notified Body
A government-sanctioned organization that can register and/or certify a quality system or product and determine that the system or product meets European Union requirements.

Placing on the Market
Making available in return for payment or free of charge of a device other than a device intended for clinical investigations, with a view to distribution and/or on the Community market regardless of whether it is new or refurbished.

Putting Into Service
The stage at which a medical device is ready for use on the European Union market for the first time for its intended purpose.

Registered/Registration
A procedure by which a registrar indicates that an organization meets the requirements of a standard or regulation.

Registrar
An accredited third party that evaluates an organization's (quality) system to verify compliance with the applicable requirements.

Reusable Surgical Instrument
An instrument intended for surgical use by cutting, drilling, sawing, scratching, scraping, clamping, retracting, clipping or similar procedures without

connection to any active medical device and that can be reused after appropriate procedures have been performed.

Short-Term Device
A device normally intended for continuous use for not more than 30 days.

Surgically Invasive Device
A device that penetrates inside the body through the surface of the body, with the aid or in the context of a surgical operation.

Transient Device
A device normally intended for continuous use for less than 60 minutes.

Transition Period
The period of time between the inception date and the enforcement date of a directive.

Index